Holiday Games and Activities

Barbara Wnek, MEd
Ferguson-Florissant School District
Florissant, Missouri

Human Kinetics Books

Library of Congress Cataloging-in-Publication Data

Wnek, Barbara, 1949-
    Holiday games and activities / Barbara Wnek.
        p.   cm
    ISBN 0-87322-355-1
    1. Physical fitness for children—Study and teaching (Elementary)-
-United States.   2. Games—United states.   3. Holidays—United
States.   I. Title.
GV443.W58   1992
372.86'0973—dc20   91-31381
                                                                   CIP

ISBN: 0-87322-355-1

Acquisitions Editor: Rick Frey, PhD; Developmental Editor: Holly Gilly; Assistant Editors: Laura Bofinger, Elizabeth Bridgett, and Moyra Knight; Copyeditor: Anne Dueweke; Proofreader: Myla Smith; Production Director: Ernie Noa; Typesetter: Sandra Meier; Text Design: Keith Blomberg; Text Layout: Denise Lowry; Cover Design: Jack Davis; Illustrations: Cindy Butler and Gretchen Walters; Printer: Versa Press

Human Kinetics books are available at special discounts for bulk purchase for sales promotions, premiums, fund-raising, or educational use. Special editions or book excerpts can also be created to specification. For details, contact the Special Sales Manager at Human Kinetics.

Printed in the United States of America   10 9 8 7 6 5 4 3 2

Human Kinetics Books
A Division of Human Kinetics Publishers
Box 5076, Champaign, IL 61825-5076
1-800-747-4457

Canada: Human Kinetics Publishers, Box 24040, Windsor, ON N8Y 4Y9
1-800-465-7301 (in Canada only)

Europe: Human Kinetics Publishers (Europe) Ltd., P.O. Box IW14,
Leeds LS16 6TR, England
0532-781708

Australia: Human Kinetics Publishers, P.O. Box 80, Kingswood 5062,
South Australia
618-374-0433

New Zealand: Human Kinetics Publishers, P.O. Box 105-231, Auckland 1
(09) 309-2259

130642

Contents

Chapter 4—DECEMBER/JANUARY: Winter, Christmas, and   63
Hanukkah

Chapter 5—FEBRUARY: Valentine's Day, Presidents' Day   87
and Groundhog Day

Chapter 6—MARCH: St. Patrick's Day   103

Acknowledgments

It's time to celebrate the completion of this book by having a holiday theme costume party. Everyone must wear a costume relating to a holiday of his or her choice. Sounds like a great way to thank all of the wonderful people who have helped me make this book a reality.

Special thanks go to Dr. Kathleen M. Haywood, professor of education, University of Missouri–St. Louis, for introducing me to Human Kinetics Publishers, answering my numerous questions, and reviewing the manuscript and artwork. Special thanks also go to Dr. Tom Loughrey, associate professor of physical education, University of Missouri–St. Louis, for referring me to the Ferguson-Florissant School District, in Florissant, Missouri, where this book began.

I would also like to thank Dr. Joyce Espiritu, coordinator of health and physical education for the Ferguson-Florissant School District, who gave me the opportunity to start writing the activities in this book for the physical education teachers. And thanks to Sandy Drey for typing them.

Many thanks also to Dr. Bruce Clark, exercise physiologist, chairperson and associate professor of physical education, University of Missouri–St. Louis, for the extra "muscle" he gave to the exercises for the book.

Thanks to Robin Hilliar, teacher at Airport School, for generously letting me use her computer when I didn't have mine. I wouldn't have made my deadline without it.

Thousands of thank yous go to all of the wonderful children who inspired me through the years to create the activities in this book.

Finally, I acknowledge the following schools and people for allowing me to develop and express my creativity throughout my years of teaching: The Ferguson-Florissant School District, Florissant, Missouri; The New City School, St. Louis, Missouri (extra thanks for letting me wear costumes for all of the special activities); The St. Louis Public Schools; Beverly Berla, executive director of The Gifted Resource Council; and Susan C. Flesch, program director of The Gifted Resource Council.

To Sophie Wnek, my mother, who has always provided me with encouragement and support and is always there for me, especially when it comes to my education. Thanks, Mom!

Preface

"When are they coming?" "Are they coming today?" "Will we get to do that?" "That was really fun!" "Can we do it again?"

These are quotes from my students referring to "Escape From the Spiders," an obstacle course activity explained in this book. I can hardly get out of my car in the morning before being greeted with questions like these. What a great way to start the day! It tells me that my students look forward to coming to physical education class and really enjoy themselves. I look forward to teaching my new ideas, too. The classroom teachers are always curious to know what I'll be up to next, especially when I walk into a staff meeting wearing my spider headband on "Escape From the Spiders" day. The anticipation and excitement the activities in this book can create will make the teaching-learning process beneficial for everyone involved. Another student asked, "Are we going to flip today?" referring to our "I Love P.E." Valentine's Day tumbling show. My students have flipped all right—over physical education. The enthusiasm created by the activities in this book is contagious, so get ready!

The school year is filled with holidays. This book presents physical fitness activities, skills, games, and rhythm and dance activities for kindergarten through sixth grade, in a holiday or seasonal theme. Most of the activities can easily be adapted for various grade or skill levels and fit into any curriculum. Holiday-related activities will bring excitement to your physical education classes, motivate your students, and provide enjoyable educational experiences. The activities in this book all have a holiday or seasonal theme. For example, "Turkey Trot" is a physical fitness circuit training course in which students can earn a paper feather with their name on it to add to the "well-done" turkey bulletin board. "Escape From the Spiders" is an obstacle course in which students must avoid touching the paper spiders they encounter along the way. If they complete the course correctly they receive a certificate that says, "I Escaped From the Spiders in Physical Education Class." "Put the Muscles on the Principal" is an exercise game in which students match the exercises performed and the muscles used. The "Blizzard" is a creative, manipulative dance activity using sheets of plastic trash bags. "Ghost Throwing" is one of the Halloween skills stations in which handkerchief ghosts are thrown instead of balls or beanbags. "Scrambled Eggs" is an Easter relay race in which the teams work together to unscramble the pieces of a paper Easter egg. "Hot Weather Water Tag" is a chasing and fleeing game in which students get "tagged" by getting a small amount of water thrown on them. Be sure to read the How to Use This Book section that follows so you will be able to present the activities as effectively as possible.

For some of the activities you will need to make a few signs or pictures. This may sound like extra work, but we all know that teachers are always doing extra things for the students. Seeing the students learning and having fun is well worth the effort.

I hope these brief descriptions have made you say to yourself, "That sounds like fun," or "I bet my students would enjoy that!" They *are* fun and the students love them, and there are many, many more included in this book. Have fun!

How to Use This Book

It is important that you take a few minutes to read the information that follows so you can effectively use the games and activities to motivate and excite your students.

HOW THE BOOK IS ORGANIZED

The book is divided thematically into eight chapters that encompass the seasons and holidays of the school year, beginning with September and ending with May/June (December and January are also combined to include the winter and holiday season). Each chapter contains the following activities:

- A circuit training course with a motivational bulletin board idea that includes using award certificates to acknowledge student effort and participation
- A challenging obstacle course with award certificates
- Skill lessons or skill practice stations
- Various types of games, including chasing and fleeing games, muscle-name learning games, and relay races
- Rhythm and dance activities, including creative movement and aerobic activities
- Other special fun activities

The explanations for each of the preceding activities are given in a format that shows at a glance the important things you need to know to present the activity to your class. Each activity has an explanatory illustration and is presented with the following information:

- Activity Title—Gives the activity a fun name to create excitement among the students.
- Quick Description—Briefly describes the activity.
- Appropriate Grades—Tells what grade levels the activity is most successful with.
- Activity Goals—Briefly describes intended outcomes of the activities for the students.

- Space Required—Tells what type of space is most suitable for the activity.
- Key Skills—Lists the skills that are emphasized in the activity.
- Equipment and Preparation—Tells what equipment is needed for the activity and explains any pre-activity preparation that might be necessary. The equipment needs are noted in boldface type so you can do a quick and easy inventory before you begin the activity.
- Activity Procedure—Explains how to conduct the activity. (See the next section for more complete information on procedures for circuit training courses, obstacle courses, and skill stations.)
- Safety Considerations—Alerts you to potential safety concerns specific to each activity.
- Adaptation Suggestions—Gives ideas about how the activity may be used in various situations.
- Teaching Hints—Includes helpful suggestions to make the activity proceed smoothly.

HOW TO USE THE APPENDIX

The appendix includes patterns for the awards for the circuit training and obstacle course activities. It also contains patterns for other materials used in the activities. You can reproduce these materials as needed.

HOW TO STRUCTURE CLASSES

The activities in the book can be used individually, or you can combine them to encompass an entire class period. For example, the activities should be preceded by a warm-up. The 10-minute physical fitness exercise circuit training course for a given season can be repeated each time the class meets. Skill station work could be done next, and, if time permits, a game or rhythmic activity could follow. The age, skill level, and needs of your students will determine the amount of time necessary for each activity.

HOW TO CONDUCT THE CIRCUIT TRAINING COURSE, OBSTACLE COURSE, AND SKILL STATION ACTIVITIES

The procedures for conducting the circuit training courses, obstacle courses, and skill stations are basically the same for each season. The following information should be used each time you prepare for one of those activities.

Circuit Training Courses

The circuit training courses require the students to perform flexibility or muscular strength and endurance exercises. Most of the exercises required should be familiar to physical educators. However, if you'd like to substitute exercises for the ones suggested, or if you're unfamiliar with the proper techniques for the exercises suggested, I encourage you to consult the following resources:

Developmental Movement Exercises for Children (1982) by David Gallahue, published by Macmillan, New York, NY.

Children Moving: A Teacher's Guide to Developing a Successful Physical Education Program (2nd ed.) (1987) by George Graham and Shirley Holt/Hale, published by Mayfield, Mountainview, CA.

More Fitness Exercises for Children by Jim Stillwell and Jerry Stockard, distributed by Great Activities Publishing Company, Durham, NC.

To make the circuit training courses run smoothly, divide the class evenly among the stations. When you give the signal, students perform the exercise at the station to which they are assigned as many times as they can or for as long as they can. Allow 10 to 20 seconds at each station. When the time limit is up for the first station, blow a whistle. This is the signal for the students to change stations. The students jog or perform another locomotor skill for one complete lap, moving counterclockwise and passing the station they just completed to proceed to the next station. Then they perform the exercise at the next station until the whistle blows for them to jog another lap. A completed course means that a student has performed all of the exercises at the stations correctly and has jogged all of the laps. Students earn awards each time they complete the circuit training course. The awards can be presented at the end of class. Student helpers can attach the awards to the wall or bulletin board for you to save time.

When selecting exercises for the courses, remember to alternate the major muscle groups being exercised. Emphasize correct form while the students are performing the exercises. Also emphasize that the students jog or perform another locomotor skill at an even pace when doing laps. They should not race when it is time to change stations. Tell students to place hand weights, ropes, or other equipment away from the jogging area when they are finished using them.

Obstacle Courses

Divide the class into as many groups as there are activities in the obstacle course. Start each group on a different activity. Pair students. One of the pair participates in the course while the other watches to ensure that the skills are being performed correctly and to count the number of obstacles touched. The first group of students starts on your signal. When these students finish the course, they should be at the same place as when they started. Partners change places and wait for the signal. Then the remainder of the class performs the obstacle course in the same manner as the first group did.

Emphasize that the obstacle course is not a race. Accidents happen when children rush through activities. Stress correct form and avoiding obstacles. Also stress keeping some space between the students. Tell students if a traffic jam occurs to please wait patiently and not to rush the performers.

Spread the obstacle course out as much as possible. Keep scooterboards under control at all times. Stress that the scooterboards used in some of the obstacle courses are not skateboards and students may not stand up on them. Students should not roll scooterboards across the floor when there is no one on them because they might hit someone. Students should also keep fingers, long hair, and necklaces away from the wheels.

Be sure to place an adequate number of mats around equipment such as the balance beam, horizontal ladder, and cargo net.

Skills Stations

Divide the class evenly among the stations. Put students in the order in which they will take their turns to prevent arguing about who is first. Tell them to keep this order for all of the stations. Line up students at each station in numerical order. Designate the number of tries that each student may take each time his or her turn comes up. The first student in each group takes a turn. Then the second student in each group takes a turn, and so on. Students continue to take turns at the first station until you give the signal for them to stop. Each group then rotates to the next station in numerical order. The stations should be numbered to prevent confusion. The student taking a turn when the stop signal is given becomes the first turn-taker at the next station. The other students line up in numerical order behind that student. This way everyone gets an equal number of turns. Give the stop signal when you see that all of the students have had at least one turn at their station. The students may keep score at the skill stations if desired.

Leave ample space between the stations and ensure that students waiting for a turn keep a safe distance from the student who is performing.

Station work is a good opportunity to give individual help, but watch for students who have difficulty staying on task. Some students need more time to adjust to the freedom involved in station work.

HOW TO PREPARE MATERIALS

Several of the activities require that you make signs or other visual aids. The signs and materials should be colorful, and large enough for students to read. Exercise signs should describe or illustrate the exercise to be performed, any important points necessary for execution, and safety precautions as appropriate. Older students love to help prepare these materials. Laminating the signs and materials will protect them, and you will be able to use them year after year.

Chapter 1

SEPTEMBER

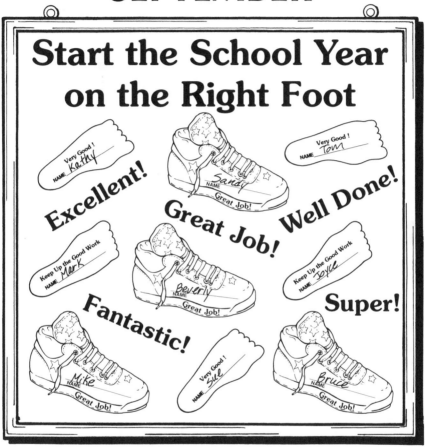

Start the School Year on the Right Foot

BACK TO SCHOOL

Start the School Year on the Right Foot

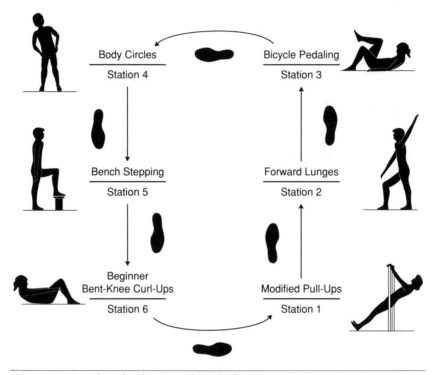

Figure 1.1 Start the school year on the right foot.

QUICK DESCRIPTION
Physical fitness exercise circuit training course (Figure 1.1)

APPROPRIATE GRADES
K-6

ACTIVITY GOALS
To improve physical fitness levels, especially muscular strength and endurance and cardiovascular endurance, by motivating the students to put more effort into the physical fitness exercises

SPACE REQUIRED
Gymnasium, track, or large outside area

KEY SKILLS

The September circuit training course emphasizes the following skills:

- Arm and shoulder strength and endurance (modified pull-ups)
- Leg strength and endurance (forward lunges, bench stepping)
- Abdominal strength (bicycle pedaling, beginner bent-knee curl-ups)
- Trunk strength (body circles)
- Cardiovascular endurance (walking, jogging)

EQUIPMENT AND PREPARATION

Start this circuit training course at the beginning of the school year in September. For the sample circuit training course, construct **7 signs**, one for each of the six exercise stations and one that says "Start the School Year on the Right Foot." The station signs should be "Modified Pull-Ups," "Forward Lunges," "Bicycle Pedaling," "Body Circles," "Bench Stepping," and "Beginner Bent-Knee Curl-Ups." Reproduce enough **"I Started the School Year on the Right Foot" certificates** (Figure A.1a in the appendix) and paper **"footnotes"** (Figure A.1b in the appendix) for everyone in your class. Make some extra **footprints** to tape to the floor for the students to follow when they change stations.

Before the lesson, tape or otherwise attach the "I Started the School Year on the Right Foot" sign to a wall or bulletin board where everyone can see it, and set up the exercise stations. You will need **modified pull-up bars** and **benches or folded mats** about 12 inches high to accommodate about six students for each station.

Build excitement and interest by putting up signs around the school on the first day that say "Start the School Year on the Right Foot" or "You Can Perform Amazing Feats in Physical Education Class!"

ACTIVITY PROCEDURE

Review the activity procedures for circuit training courses on page xii. Because this is the beginning of the school year, it will take time to teach the students the correct way to perform the flexibility and strength and endurance exercises. Make sure all students are performing them correctly before they participate in the circuit training course. This way you won't have to make many corrections or reteach the exercises later.

Because this is early in the year, have the students walk through the changing procedure for the circuit training course. Once the routine is established, students can jog the laps instead of walking.

Students earn an "I Started the School Year on the Right Foot" certificate the first time they correctly complete the course in one class period, and a paper "footnote" any time after that to put up on the wall or bulletin board.

SAFETY CONSIDERATIONS

Emphasize correct form while the students are performing the exercises. Make sure that all students are performing them correctly.

ADAPTATION SUGGESTIONS

The size of the circuit can be reduced at the beginning of the year and increased as the year progresses. The exercises and aerobic activities can be adapted to the individual needs of the children.

TEACHING HINTS

Take as much time as you need at the beginning of the school year to make sure all students understand procedures and routines, and are performing the activities correctly. The rest of the school year will proceed more smoothly if you take this time now.

A section of the wall in the gym can be called "Amazing Feats." You can post neat things that the students do relating to physical education either during school or in their free time.

The Road of Rules

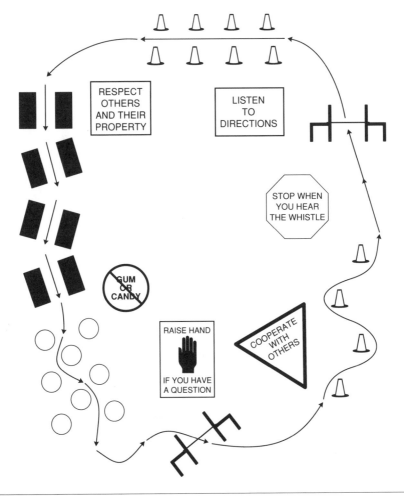

RESPECT
OTHERS
AND THEIR
PROPERTY

LISTEN
TO
DIRECTIONS

STOP WHEN
YOU HEAR
THE WHISTLE

GUM
OR
CANDY

RAISE HAND

IF YOU HAVE
A QUESTION

COOPERATE
WITH
OTHERS

Figure 1.2 The road of rules.

QUICK DESCRIPTION
Obstacle course (Figure 1.2)

APPROPRIATE GRADES
K-6

ACTIVITY GOALS
To complete the skills in the obstacle course correctly, to improve arm and leg strength and endurance, and to learn physical education class rules

SPACE REQUIRED

Gymnasium

KEY SKILLS

Bodily control in maneuvering scooterboard through obstacles while sitting or lying in a prone (face down) position; learning and following class rules

EQUIPMENT AND PREPARATION

Construct **class rule signs** that resemble traffic signs. Here are some examples:

- Walk, don't speed, into the gym.
- Do not eat or chew gum.
- Raise your hand if you have a question.
- When the whistle blows, stop, look at the teacher, and listen.
- Yield—cooperate with other students.
- Respect others and their property.

Reproduce enough **"I Know the Rules" certificates** (Figure A.2 in the appendix) for everyone in your class.

Before the lesson, set up the obstacle course to resemble a street, with obstacles to maneuver through and under while sitting or lying on a scooterboard. Make instruction signs for each obstacle in the course. You will need **1 scooterboard** for each pair of students, a large number of **traffic cones** or other obstacles, **8 hoops or tires, 4 chairs, 2 sticks** about 6 feet long, and enough **tumbling mats** to make obstacles. Attach the rule signs to traffic cones and place them along the course for the students to read as they go along.

ACTIVITY PROCEDURE

Review the activity procedures for obstacle courses on page xiii. Explain the obstacle course to the class. All students participating in the obstacle course receive an "I Know the Rules" certificate with the class rules printed on it. This will help reinforce learning the class rules. Review the rules as you pass out the certificates at the end of class.

These are the activities in the sample course:

- traveling through traffic cones in a prone position with hands leading
- traveling under stick while sitting with feet leading
- traveling between traffic cones while sitting backwards
- traveling between mats while sitting with feet leading

- traveling through hoops or tires in a prone position with hands leading
- traveling under stick in a prone position with feet leading

SAFETY CONSIDERATIONS

To avoid accidents, limit the number of scooterboards moving through the course at one time. Emphasize that students must start on the signal and stop when they complete the course. Tell the students that the class rules are mainly for safety and to make maximum use of class time.

ADAPTATION SUGGESTIONS

You may not want younger children to use scooterboards so soon in the school year. Instead, they can pretend they are driving through the obstacle course while walking.

TEACHING HINTS

If students don't follow class rules give them violation "tickets" and send them to time-out. Have the student who is not performing be a "traffic patroller" to read out the class rule signs as they are approached.

September Remember Skills Stations

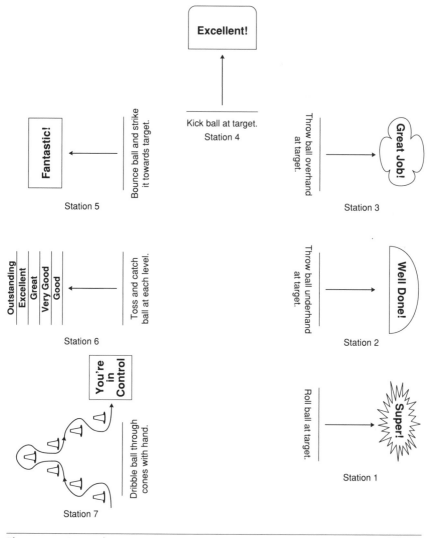

Figure 1.3 September remember.

QUICK DESCRIPTION
Ball-handling skills stations with positive message targets (Figure 1.3)

APPROPRIATE GRADES
K-6

ACTIVITY GOALS

To review various ball-handling skills from the previous year and perform them correctly

SPACE REQUIRED

Gymnasium

KEY SKILLS

Rolling, underhand throwing, overhand throwing, catching, bouncing, kicking, and striking

EQUIPMENT AND PREPARATION

Construct **5 signs** to use as targets. Write positive messages on the signs such as "Great Job," "Excellent," "Super," "Well Done," and "Fantastic." You will also need **5 smaller strips of paper** with positive messages, each one better than the last. The signs could say "Good," "Very Good," "Great," "Excellent," and "Outstanding." These signs are for tossing to oneself and catching. Make **a sign** for the bouncing station that says "You're in Control."

Set up the stations in the gym. You will need various types of **balls** (playground, soccer, basketball, tennis, softball) and **7 traffic cones**.

ACTIVITY PROCEDURE

Review the activity procedures for skills stations on page xiv. Explain each station to the class.

Station Description

- Students roll the ball at the "Super" sign.
- Students throw the ball underhand at the "Well Done" sign.
- Students throw the ball overhand at the "Great Job" sign.
- Students kick the ball at the "Excellent" sign.
- Students bounce the ball and strike it towards the "Fantastic" sign.

- Students toss the ball to the first level (Good) and catch it, then toss the ball to the second level (Very Good) and catch it. Repeat this procedure at the third level (Great), fourth level (Excellent), and fifth level (Outstanding). If a student misses the catch before getting to the fifth level, his or her turn is over and the next student begins.

- Students bounce (dribble) the ball through the cones without missing or without hitting the cones. If they do it correctly they are "in control." (Stress control.)

SAFETY CONSIDERATIONS

Leave ample space between stations. Tell students to be careful to avoid collisions when retrieving balls.

ADAPTATION SUGGESTIONS

Older students can use softballs for the target throws, soccer balls for the kicking, and basketballs for the bouncing (dribbling).

TEACHING HINTS

Review the correct way to perform the skills before the students participate at the stations.

Footsies

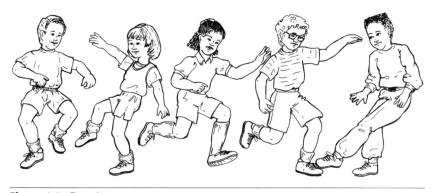

Figure 1.4 Footsies.

QUICK DESCRIPTION

A chasing and fleeing game (Figure 1.4)

APPROPRIATE GRADES

K-6

ACTIVITY GOALS

To demonstrate bodily control and to follow game rules and safety rules in a game situation

SPACE REQUIRED

Gymnasium or outside area with marked boundaries

KEY SKILLS

Running, chasing, fleeing, dodging, and tagging safely; and developing honesty and good sportsmanship

EQUIPMENT AND PREPARATION

None, unless you need to mark off boundaries.

ACTIVITY PROCEDURE

Footsies is a game of tag in which everyone is a chaser and is being chased simultaneously. When the start signal is given students try to lightly tap as many of the other players' feet as possible, while preventing their own feet from being tapped. Players may not hold other players to tag them. Only the feet may be used.

SAFETY CONSIDERATIONS

Emphasize that students tap lightly when tagging the other players. Clear the playing area of dangerous objects and hazards, and keep the boundary lines away from walls or fences to avoid accidents. Also stress that the students watch where they are running at all times to avoid collisions.

ADAPTATION SUGGESTIONS

This game can be used as a simple aerobic warm-up activity, or students can keep their own score by subtracting the number of times their own feet were tapped from the number of other players' feet they tapped.

Younger children will enjoy playing the game without keeping score. Older children, being more competitive, will prefer to keep score. At the end of the game, ask students how many points they earned.

TEACHING HINTS

Tell students that they must stay on their feet during the game and not fall down purposely to avoid being tagged.

Put the Muscles on the Principal

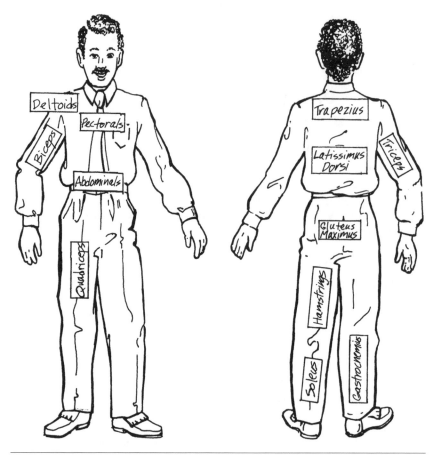

Figure 1.5 Put the muscles on the principal.

QUICK DESCRIPTION
An exercise and muscle-name learning game (Figure 1.5)

APPROPRIATE GRADES
K-6

ACTIVITY GOALS
To perform exercises correctly and to name and locate muscles used during the exercises

SPACE REQUIRED
Gymnasium or large classroom

KEY SKILLS

Flexibility and strengthening exercises and knowledge of major muscle groups used during the exercises

EQUIPMENT AND PREPARATION

You will need **2 pieces of butcherblock or other paper** about 7 feet long and 3 feet wide (large enough for the outline of an adult's body), **a pencil, a marker,** and **a human body muscle chart.** Make arrangements for the principal to come to your class for a few minutes to have his or her body outlined on the paper. The students really enjoy this. To complete the body, ask the principal for a **photograph** of him- or herself and enlarge it on the copy machine so that the face is life-size. Attach it to the body outline when the principal comes to your class.

You will also need to make **exercise/muscle cards.** This can be done by writing flexibility or strength and endurance exercises, and muscles used, on index cards and laminating them. Tape a piece of plastic (laminating plastic will work fine) to each of the different muscle locations on the paper outline so the cards can be attached and removed easily without tearing the outline. Putty-like picture-to-wall adhesive works better than masking tape because the cards can be removed easily.

ACTIVITY PROCEDURE

When the principal comes to your class, have the two large pieces of paper taped to a wall where the whole class can see them. Ask the principal to stand with his or her back to the paper. Choose a student to outline the body. Have a stool or bench handy in case the student has a difficult time reaching to the height of the principal. Use pencil first and go over it in marker later. (I don't think your principal would appreciate marker on his or her clothes.) Tape the photocopied photograph where the face should be. Then have the principal turn around and face the paper and choose another student to trace the rear view outline.

Select the exercise/muscle cards you are going to use. Give the name of the exercise, explain and demonstrate the correct way to perform the exercise, and give any safety precautions. Tell the students which muscle group is being exercised and show them where it is located on the muscle chart. Choose a student to attach the exercise/muscle card to the outline of the principal in the correct place. Then have the class perform the exercise, and make corrections as necessary.

Repeat this procedure for all of the exercises you have selected.

SAFETY CONSIDERATIONS

Stress correct form while performing all the exercises and mention any safety precautions.

ADAPTATION SUGGESTIONS

Younger students can play put the body parts on the principal (make cards with the names of body parts on them), and then progress to the names of the muscles.

TEACHING HINTS

Take time at the beginning of the school year to make sure all the students are performing the exercises correctly. This will save time making corrections or reteaching them later.

Because this is the beginning of the school year, teach and lead the exercises for a while to make sure all students are performing them correctly. Students can lead the exercises in the future.

You can repeat this activity in December. Just substitute a Santa cut-out for the principal.

Muscle or Body-Part Targets

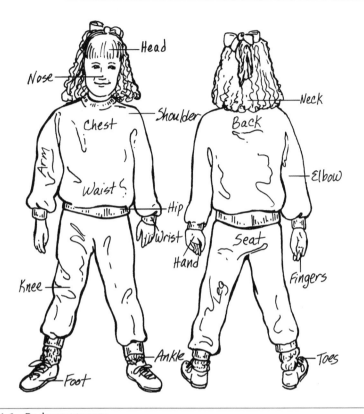

Figure 1.6 Body-part targets.

QUICK DESCRIPTION

Underhand or overhand throwing game (Figures 1.5, muscle target on page 12, and Figure 1.6)

APPROPRIATE GRADES

K-6

ACTIVITY GOALS

To improve form and accuracy when performing the underhand or overhand throw and to reinforce learning the names and locations of the muscles or body parts

SPACE REQUIRED

Gymnasium

KEY SKILLS

Underhand throwing, overhand throwing, and demonstrating knowledge of muscles or body parts and their locations

EQUIPMENT AND PREPARATION

It may take one class period for the students to make the targets. You will need **pieces of butcherblock or other paper** large enough to outline a student's body; **pencils and markers; a human body muscle chart; masking tape**; and **sponge balls, fleece balls, or beanbags**. Each student can have their own piece of paper, two students can share one piece of paper (one can be the front view and the other the rear view), or a small group of students can use one piece of paper (they will have to choose whose body will be outlined).

ACTIVITY PROCEDURE

Divide the students into groups according to the number of targets you want. For example, if you have a class of 24 students and you want eight targets, divide the class into groups of three. Give each group a piece of paper, a pencil, and a marker. One of the students can be outlined for the front view, one for the rear view, and one student can do the outlining. They can use both sides of the paper, one for the front view and the other for the rear view. When the students are finished outlining, call out the names of different muscles or body parts. Have the students point to the location of the muscles or body part on the outline and write the name of the muscle or body part in the correct place. Remember to do both front and rear views. When the outlines are completed, have students tape them to the wall, either with the front or rear view showing. Spread them out so there is ample room between the targets. Students will also need a piece of masking tape on the floor to stand behind when they throw at the targets.

To play the game, a student stands behind the restraining line and names one of the muscles or body parts on the outline. Using the designated type of throw (underhand or overhand), the student throws at the target. If the student hits the targeted muscle or body part, he or she gets one point. If the student misses the targeted muscle or body part, no point is earned. Then the second and third students in the group take their turns in the same manner.

SAFETY CONSIDERATIONS

Leave plenty of space between the targets.

ADAPTATION SUGGESTIONS

Younger children can throw at the different parts of the body, and then progress to the names and locations of the muscles.

TEACHING HINTS

The body outline may be reversed during the game so the other muscles or body parts are included. Students can keep their own record of the number of times they hit the muscle or body part they are aiming for out of the number of turns they have, or students in the group can compete against one another.

Stress correct throwing form. Students should have been given previous instruction in the underhand and overhand throws. Review the skills with them before they use the body targets.

Spelling Relays

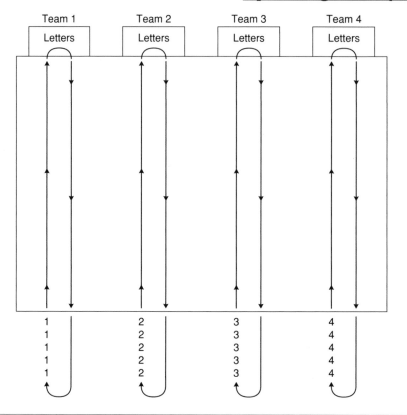

Figure 1.7 Spelling relays.

QUICK DESCRIPTION

Spelling incorporated into relay races (Figure 1.7)

APPROPRIATE GRADES

K-6

ACTIVITY GOALS

To work cooperatively as part of a team to spell words correctly and to perform various locomotor skills correctly

SPACE REQUIRED

Gymnasium

KEY SKILLS

Various locomotor movements such as running, galloping, skipping, and animal walks; cooperating in a team game; obeying the rules of a game; demonstrating safety rules while playing a game; and spelling correctly

EQUIPMENT AND PREPARATION

Decide which words to use. You can use **physical education terms** or ask a classroom teacher for a **spelling list**. In large letters, print each word on paper, photocopy it, and cut the letters apart. The number of copies you make will depend on the number of relay teams. You will need **a small box or container** for each team to put the letters in (a turned-over flying disc works fine).

ACTIVITY PROCEDURE

Explain the relay race to the class. Divide the class as evenly as possible into relay teams. Arrange the teams in single-file lines at one end of the gym behind a starting line. You can make the line with masking tape if there is no line painted on the gym floor. At the other end of the gym, place a container with the letters to a word inside, even with each team.

On the signal, the first student in each line performs the designated locomotor skill to the container, takes one letter from the container, returns to the starting line, and tags right hands with the next team member. This procedure continues until all of the letters have been retrieved. As the race is in progress, team members work together to spell the word correctly. The first team that spells the word correctly is the winner.

SAFETY CONSIDERATIONS

Place the starting line and containers a safe distance from walls to avoid accidents.

ADAPTATION SUGGESTIONS

You can vary the difficulty of the spelling. For younger children, print the word on a separate piece of paper so they can match the letters to the word. To make it more difficult, say the word and spell it, or just say the word. The most difficult would be not to say what the word is. The students would have to unscramble the letters to find out. You can also vary the locomotor skills according to ability.

TEACHING HINTS

Make sure each team knows its container so there is no confusion when the race starts. It's a good idea to walk each team through the race procedure first. Choose words with enough letters so that every student on a team gets at least one turn.

In the excitement of the race, watch for students who grab more than one letter out of the container.

Creative Aerobics

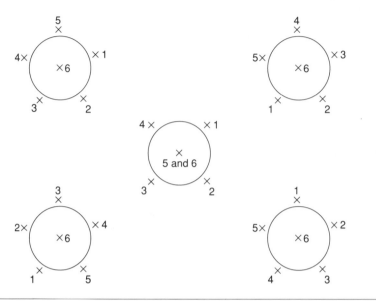

Figure 1.8 Creative aerobics.

QUICK DESCRIPTION
Student-led aerobic exercise (Figure 1.8)

APPROPRIATE GRADES
K-6

ACTIVITY GOALS
To choose an aerobic movement and effectively lead a small group in performing it to music

SPACE REQUIRED
Gymnasium

KEY SKILLS
Moving aerobically to the rhythm of the music and leading a group

EQUIPMENT AND PREPARATION
Students should have had some previous experience with aerobic movement or dancing to music. You will need **a record or cassette player** and **a piece of music** that will motivate the students to move aerobically. My students really enjoy the song "Tequila" (The Champs, Masters International Inc.).

ACTIVITY PROCEDURE

Divide the class into groups with a similar number of students in each group. Assign the students in each group a number. For a group that has fewer students, assign one student two numbers. Play part of the music so the students can become familiar with it. Have each group of students make a circle. Then call out a number. The student with this number in each group stands in the center of the circle. This student is the first exercise leader. When the music begins, the leaders perform an aerobic movement to the music. The other students perform the same movement as their leader until you call another number. Then the student in each group with the second number becomes the exercise leader. This continues until all the numbers have been called and all students have had a chance to lead. Stress continuous movement. Have the students walk around the gym for a few minutes to cool down.

SAFETY CONSIDERATIONS

When you make the circles, leave plenty of space between the students. Tell the students they must stay on their feet for this activity.

ADAPTATION SUGGESTIONS

You may want to use different types of music for various age groups.

TEACHING HINTS

If some students are a bit shy or are having trouble thinking of a movement, give them some suggestions.

Chapter 2

OCTOBER

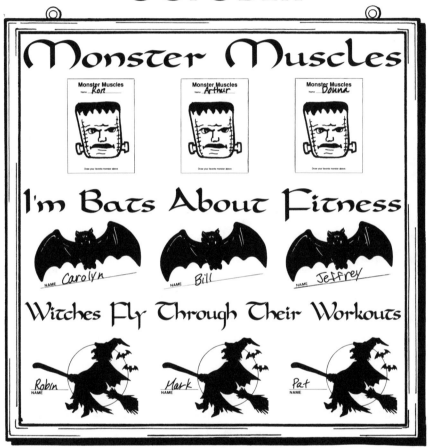

HALLOWEEN

Monster Muscles, I'm Bats About Fitness, and Witches Fly Through Their Workouts

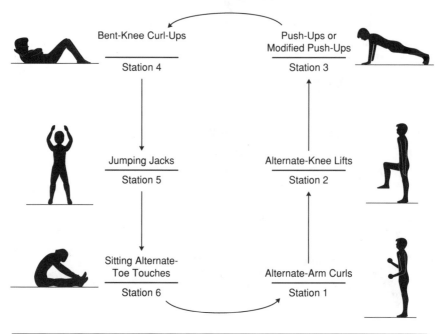

Figure 2.1 Monster muscles, I'm bats about fitness, and witches fly through their workouts.

QUICK DESCRIPTION

Physical fitness exercise circuit training course (Figure 2.1)

APPROPRIATE GRADES

K-6

ACTIVITY GOALS

To improve physical fitness levels, especially muscular strength and endurance and cardiovascular endurance, by motivating students to put more effort into the physical fitness exercises

SPACE REQUIRED

Gymnasium, track, or large outside area

KEY SKILLS

The Halloween circuit training course emphasizes the following skills:

- Arm strength and endurance (alternate-arm curls with hand weights)
- Leg strength and endurance (alternate-knee lifts)
- Arm and shoulder-girdle strength and endurance (push-ups or modified push-ups)
- Abdominal strength and endurance (bent-knee curl-ups)
- General body conditioning (jumping jacks)
- Trunk strength (sitting alternate-toe touches)
- Cardiovascular endurance (jogging)

EQUIPMENT AND PREPARATION

Start this circuit training course at the beginning of October. Construct **9 signs**, one for each of the six exercise stations plus three more that say "Monster Muscles," "I'm Bats About Fitness," and "Witches Fly Through Their Workouts." The station signs should be "Alternate-Arm Curls," "Alternate-Knee Lifts," "Push-Ups or Modified Push-Ups," "Bent-Knee Curl-Ups With a Twist," "Jumping Jacks," and "Sitting Alternate-Toe Touches." Reproduce enough **"Monster Muscle" certificates** (Figure A.3a in the appendix), **bats** (Figure A.3b in the appendix), and **witches' brooms** (Figure A.3c in the appendix) for everyone in your class.

Attach the other three signs to a prominent wall or bulletin board, and set up the stations. You will need **6 traffic cones** and **4 or 5 pairs of 1- to 3-pound hand weights**. If you plan to have Halloween music, you will need **a record or cassette player** and **a piece of music**.

Build excitement and interest by putting up signs around the school about a week before you schedule the course that say "Do You Have Monster Muscles?" "Are You Bats About Fitness?" or "Are You a Witch Who Flies Through a Workout?"

ACTIVITY PROCEDURE

Review the activity procedures for circuit training courses on page xii. Allow about 20 seconds at each station.

Each time students correctly complete the course, they earn the choice of a "Monster Muscles" certificate (on which they draw a picture of a monster during their free time), a paper bat with their name on it, or a paper witch's broom with their name on it. Place the certificates, bats, and witches' brooms on the wall under the corresponding sign.

SAFETY CONSIDERATIONS

Emphasize correct form while the students are performing the exercises. Tell students to place the hand weights away from the jogging area when they are finished using them.

ADAPTATION SUGGESTIONS

For the younger children, reduce the circumference of the circuit, or the jog between stations can be deleted if desired. The younger students can pretend they are bats flying through the air or witches flying on their brooms when they change stations. Other locomotor and nonlocomotor activities, such as animal walks, jumping, galloping, hopping, and skipping can be substituted for some of the exercises or for the jogging. Children with disabilities can be given appropriate movement challenges.

TEACHING HINTS

Choose exercises with which the children are already familiar. You can use cans of food in place of hand weights.

Try playing Halloween music while the children are exercising.

Escape From the Spiders

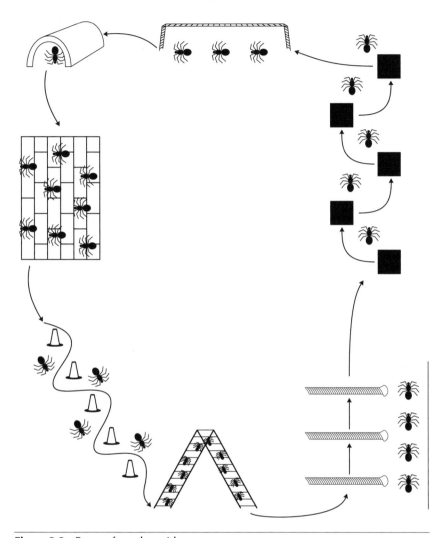

Figure 2.2 Escape from the spiders.

QUICK DESCRIPTION
Obstacle course (Figure 2.2)

APPROPRIATE GRADES
K-6

ACTIVITY GOALS
To complete the skills in the obstacle course correctly without touching any of the paper spiders

27

SPACE REQUIRED

Gymnasium

KEY SKILLS

Bodily control while performing the entire obstacle course, perceptual motor skills, traveling from one hanging rope to another, jumping from base to base, traveling while hanging on to the rungs of the horizontal ladder, maneuvering through the tunnel, climbing the cargo net, jumping with a ball between the knees, and climbing over ladders or other obstacles

EQUIPMENT AND PREPARATION

Reproduce about **30 paper spiders** (Figure A.4a in the appendix) and enough **"I Escaped From the Spider" certificates** (Figure A.4b in the appendix) for everyone in your class. The more spiders there are, the more the students enjoy it. Assemble the obstacle course and attach the spiders to various places along the course. You will need some or all of the following: **equipment for climbing such as hanging ropes, climbing ladders, horizontal ladders, and cargo nets; 4 or more rubber bases; 1 parachute draped over chairs to make a tunnel; 5 traffic cones; 1 playground ball;** and enough **mats and thick crash mats** to use around the equipment.

To motivate students, put up signs around the school about a week before the activity is scheduled that say "The Spiders Are Coming! Will You Be Able to Escape?"

ACTIVITY PROCEDURE

Review the activity procedures for obstacle courses on page xiii. Explain the obstacle course to the class. Students who complete the course correctly without touching any spiders, receive an "I Escaped From the Spiders" certificate.

These are the activities included in the sample course:

- traveling on hanging ropes without falling into the spider pit
- jumping from base to base without stepping on the spiders on the floor
- traveling along the rungs on the horizontal ladder without falling into a spider pit
- crawling through the tunnel without touching any spiders
- climbing up and down the cargo net (spider web) without touching any spiders
- jumping through the path of cones while holding a ball between the knees without stepping on any spiders
- climbing over ladders or obstacles without touching any spiders

SAFETY CONSIDERATIONS

Emphasize that the students begin on the signal and stop when they complete the course. Tell students that the rules are mainly for safety and to make maximum use of class time.

ADAPTATION SUGGESTIONS

You can vary the activities according to the skill levels of the children. For example, for younger children, move the bases closer together, limit the climbing height on the cargo net, and reduce the distance children must travel on the horizontal ladder. Adapt activities as necessary for children with disabilities.

TEACHING HINTS

Choose activities with which the students are familiar.

The student who is not performing can count the number of spiders touched by his or her partner.

Halloween Skills Stations

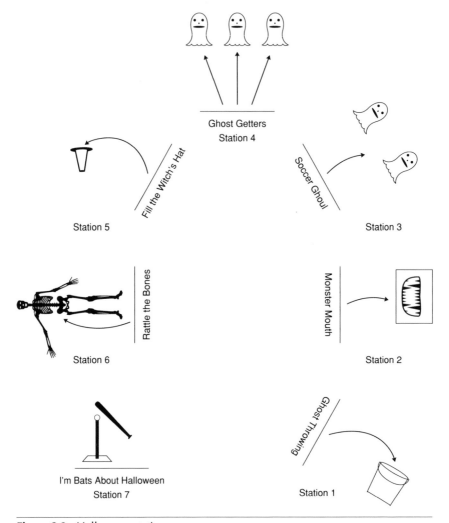

Figure 2.3 Halloween stations.

QUICK DESCRIPTION
Ball handling and striking and kicking skills stations (Figure 2.3)

APPROPRIATE GRADES
K-6

ACTIVITY GOALS
To improve form and accuracy while rolling, underhand throwing, overhand throwing, striking with a bat, and kicking

SPACE REQUIRED

Gymnasium

KEY SKILLS

Rolling, underhand throwing, overhand throwing, striking with a bat, and kicking

EQUIPMENT AND PREPARATION

This activity includes seven stations for which you will need to do the following:

- *Ghost Throwing.* Construct **a sign** that says "Ghost Throwing." Make **2 ghosts** by covering **a small ball** (styrofoam, rubber, or tennis) with **a handkerchief** and securing it with **a rubber band**. Find some type of **container** (box or trash can) to use as the target.

- *Monster Mouth.* Construct **a sign** that says "Monster Mouth." You will need **a picture of a scary mouth, a Hula Hoop, or a cardboard box** with one side cut to look like a mouth with pointed teeth, and **2 beanbags**. Students will be happy to draw the pictures for you to help you make the cardboard mouth.

- *Soccer Ghoul.* Construct **a sign** that says "Soccer Ghoul." You will need **2 pictures of a ghoul or ghost**, each attached to **a traffic cone** to make "ghoul" posts, and **a foam soccer ball**.

- *Ghost Getters.* Construct **a sign** that says "Ghost Getters." You will need **a plastic milk or bleach bottle with a scary face drawn on it or a traffic cone covered or draped with white material** (to resemble a ghost), **or an inflatable ghost**, which can be purchased at most stores that carry Halloween supplies. You will also need **2 beanbags or 2 lightweight balls** (if you are using the inflatable ghost, which could be broken by the beanbags).

- *Fill the Witch's Hat.* Construct **a sign** that says "Fill the Witch's Hat." You will need **a low basketball hoop or a traffic cone turned upside down and covered with black material** to resemble a witch's hat, and **a small playground ball or tennis ball**.

- *Rattle the Bones.* Construct **a sign** that says "Rattle the Bones." You will need **a picture of a skeleton** that can be attached to the wall **or an inflatable or plastic skeleton** that can be suspended from a bar. You will also need **2 beanbags** (if you are using a picture of a skeleton) or **2 lightweight balls** (if you are using the inflatable or plastic skeleton).

- *I'm Bats About Halloween.* Construct **a sign** that says "I'm Bats About Halloween." You will need **a batting tee, a plastic bat**, and **a lightweight ball**.

Set up the stations in the gym and attach the corresponding signs to the wall. Also mark lines on the floor with **masking tape** behind which the students must stand when taking their turns.

ACTIVITY PROCEDURE

Review the activity procedures for skills stations on page xiv. Explain each station to the class.

Station Description

- *Ghost Throwing*—Students throw the "ghosts" into the container.

- *Monster Mouth*—Students either throw beanbags into the cardboard monster mouth, through the Hula Hoop, or at the picture of the mouth.

- *Soccer Ghoul*—Students kick the soccer ball between the "ghoul" posts.

- *Ghost Getters*—Students hit the ghost with a beanbag or lightweight ball.

- *Fill the Witch's Hat*—Students make a basket or throw the ball into the cone.

- *Rattle the Bones*—Students hit the picture of the skeleton with a beanbag or try to hit the inflatable or plastic skeleton with a lightweight ball.

- *I'm Bats About Halloween*—Students hit the lightweight ball off the batting tee.

SAFETY CONSIDERATIONS

Make sure that students who are awaiting their turns are not too close to the student who is taking a turn, especially at the batting station.

ADAPTATION SUGGESTIONS

Younger students can progress from rolling balls at the targets to throwing. Be sure to lower the targets for rolling. You can substitute another activity for the batting station until the students are ready for batting. Shorten or lengthen the distance from the restraining line to the target according to skill level. Also adjust skills appropriately for children with disabilities.

TEACHING HINTS

Teach or review the skills with the students before they practice at the stations. Students can retrieve the objects after their turn and give them to the next student.

Ghost Throwing

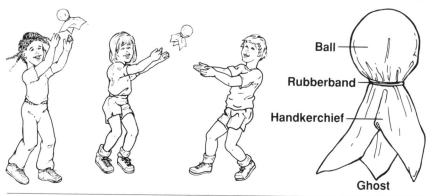

Figure 2.4 Instructions for making "ghosts" and using them.

QUICK DESCRIPTION
Manipulative activity (Figure 2.4)

APPROPRIATE GRADES
K-3

ACTIVITY GOALS
To improve skill level in tossing to self, striking, throwing underhand and overhand, and catching

SPACE REQUIRED
Gymnasium or large outside area

KEY SKILLS
Tossing to self, striking, throwing underhand and overhand, and catching

EQUIPMENT AND PREPARATION
Make a "ghost" (Figure 2.4) for each student in your class, or one ghost for every two children (then they can work in pairs and take turns). To make the ghost, cover **a small ball** (styrofoam, rubber, or tennis) with **a handkerchief** or other similar-sized piece of material, and secure with **a rubber band**. Draw a face on the material with **a permanent or laundry marker**. Styrofoam balls work well because they don't travel very far, so students won't spend time chasing the ghost. Also, if someone gets hit with a ghost accidentally, it won't hurt. These ghosts can be used year after year. The students can even help you make them.

ACTIVITY PROCEDURE

Students should practice the following activities with both their right and left hands.

Individual Activities

Tossing and Catching

- Tossing and catching while gradually increasing the height of the toss
- Tossing, clapping hands, and catching
- Tossing, turning around, and catching
- Tossing underneath the right leg and catching, and tossing underneath the left leg and catching
- Tossing from the right hand to the left hand and from the left hand to the right hand
- Tossing and catching at different levels (high, medium, and low)

Striking

- Tossing the ghost upward and striking it upward from underneath with an open hand
- Tossing the ghost upward and striking it forward with an open-hand overhead, as in volleyball
- Tossing the ghost upward and striking it forward with an open hand out to the side like a tennis forehand drive
- Striking the ghost with different body parts

Partner Activities

- Throwing underhand to a partner
- Throwing overhand to a partner
- Tossing and striking the ghost underhand to a partner
- Tossing and striking the ghost overhand to a partner
- Tossing and striking the ghost with the hand out to the side

The students can experiment with throwing the ghosts either by holding on to the ball or onto the ends of the handkerchief.

SAFETY CONSIDERATIONS

The practice area should be large enough so that students can spread out to avoid bumping into each other. Emphasize that they be careful about this, especially because their attention will be focused more on the ghosts than their classmates.

ADAPTATION SUGGESTIONS

Let students progress at their own speed. Give more challenging skills to those students who are ready. Heavier balls, such as tennis balls, make the activity more challenging. Create as many movement challenges as you like.

TEACHING HINTS

Students should have had previous experience with these skills before using the ghosts. At the beginning of the lesson, review these skills, emphasizing correct throwing and catching form.

Magic Wands

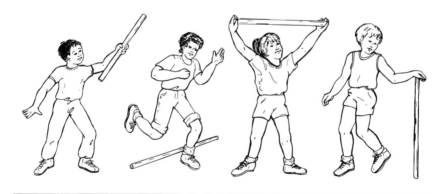

Figure 2.5 Magic wands.

QUICK DESCRIPTION

Manipulative activity with wands (Figure 2.5)

APPROPRIATE GRADES

K-6

ACTIVITY GOALS

To perform manipulative skills with wands; if music is used, to perform the skills to the beat of the music

SPACE REQUIRED

Gymnasium, large classroom or outside area

KEY SKILLS

A variety of movement challenges, exercises, and stunts can be performed with the wands. Some skills involved are bodily control, balance, locomotor and nonlocomotor skills, and flexibility. A sense of rhythm is developed if the skills are performed to music. This activity also develops creativity.

EQUIPMENT AND PREPARATION

Younger children can pretend to cast a magic spell that turns their classroom teacher into a frog. You can plan ahead of time for the teacher to wear a green paper frog mask (Figure A.5 in the appendix) when the students see him or her after physical education class. They really enjoy this.

You will need **a wand or stick** about 3 feet long, which can be either purchased or made from a 3/4-inch wooden dowel or a broom or mop handle. Ideally, you should have one wand for each student. You will also need **a record or cassette player** and **a piece of music** if you plan to use music. A variety of music can be used.

ACTIVITY PROCEDURE

Younger students can begin by playing a game of "Freeze." The students perform a movement activity as instructed and stop when you blow the whistle or say "Freeze." Students can pretend their wand is a witch's broom and fly around the room by performing different locomotor skills such as galloping, skipping, jumping, and running. The wand can also be a witch's spoon used to stir a magic brew. They can stir with both arms, or one arm at a time, making small or large circles. Here is a list of movement activities that the students can perform when pretending to cast a magic spell:

• Placing the wand on the floor and moving over and around it in a variety of ways; students can jump, hop, and make bridges over it, and walk, run, gallop, and skip around it

• Passing the wand around different body parts with the hands (waist, neck, right leg, left leg, both legs)

• Putting one end of the wand on the floor, placing one hand on top of the other end, and performing different locomotor skills (running, galloping, skipping, walking backwards, hopping) around it

- Drawing pictures or writing in the air using the wand as a pencil
- Twirling the wand in front of the body with two hands
- Balancing the wand on different body parts

- Holding the wand in front of the body with one hand on each end of it, then stepping through the space one leg at a time, and returning to the starting position without touching the wand

- Standing the wand on one end in front of the body, then letting go, turning around quickly, and grasping the wand before it falls over (students should practice with both their right and left hands)

Give students some time to create their own movements with the wands. They can work alone or with partners. Students can also create magic wand routines to music and perform them for the class. For example, one class I know made giant hot pink and yellow tissue-paper flowers that they attached to the ends of the wands. They then created a dance using the wands as props. The students made different formations on the floor such as circles and double lines. Sometimes a student held up the pink flower and at other times the yellow flower. Students also did formations in which they laid the wands on the floor and performed different movements over them. It was a very colorful and creative performance.

SAFETY CONSIDERATIONS

Students should have plenty of space to avoid accidentally hitting each other with the wands. Tell them to be very careful when performing movements over or around the wands because they could step on the wands and slip. Don't allow students to pretend that the wand is some type of weapon.

ADAPTATION SUGGESTIONS

Younger students will enjoy performing the activities to turn their teacher into a frog. Older students will prefer the more difficult stunts such as performing exercises, creating their own movements, and creating dances to the music. Older students will also prefer performing the activities to earn some other type of reward, such as free time.

TEACHING HINTS

Have the students place the wands on the floor when you are giving instructions. Otherwise some of the students will continue to practice with them or make noise by tapping them on the floor.

The wands can also be used for other activities, including "over and under" stations in obstacle courses.

Pumpkin Ball

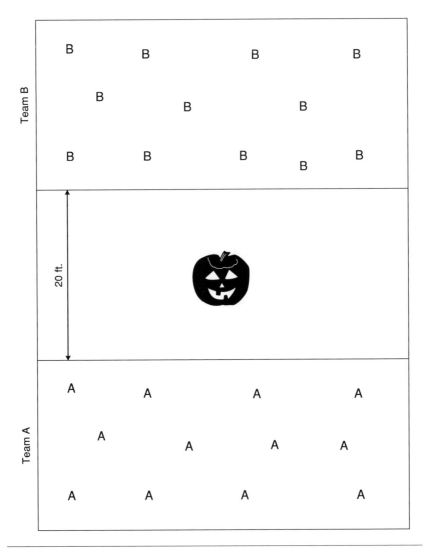

Figure 2.6 Pumpkin ball.

QUICK DESCRIPTION
Throwing-for-accuracy team game (Figure 2.6)

APPROPRIATE GRADES
K-6

ACTIVITY GOALS

To throw for accuracy in a game situation

SPACE REQUIRED

An area the size of a volleyball court with two 20-foot-long lines marked across the center of the playing area to divide the area into three zones

KEY SKILLS

Throwing, participating cooperatively in a team game, obeying the rules of a game, and demonstrating safety rules while playing a game

EQUIPMENT AND PREPARATION

Make a smiling pumpkin-like face on a **cage ball**. This can be done with any type of **tape**. You will also need **12 to 16 playground balls**. Before your class comes to the gym, put the pumpkin ball where all the students can see it. Divide the playing area into three zones as instructed under Space Required.

ACTIVITY PROCEDURE

Divide the class, as evenly as possible, into two groups. Arrange one group on one third of the playing area and the other group on the other third. Place the pumpkin ball in the center of the 20-foot-wide middle area. Divide the various types of balls equally between the two groups. Give a signal to start the game. The object of the game is to move the pumpkin ball across the line in front of the other group only by throwing balls at it. It may not be touched with the hands or pushed with a ball in a player's hands. Players may throw at the pumpkin ball only when they are behind the line that is in front of them. They may not throw from within the pumpkin-ball area. They may, however, enter the pumpkin-ball area to retrieve a ball, but must go back to their own side to throw. A group wins each time the pumpkin ball crosses the other group's line. Then the game begins again.

SAFETY CONSIDERATIONS

Tell the students to watch out for balls that rebound off the pumpkin ball. If they are very close to the pumpkin ball when they hit it, the ball they have thrown comes back very hard. Also tell them to take turns chasing the balls to prevent collisions.

ADAPTATION SUGGESTIONS

You can designate one player from each team to stay in the pumpkin-ball area to retrieve balls. If you play this way, no one else can go into the pumpkin-ball area and the ball retrievers may not touch or move the pumpkin ball.

Younger children can play in a smaller area to make it easier for them to move the pumpkin ball across the line. For the older children you can deflate the pumpkin ball slightly, which will make it more difficult to roll. A fully inflated pumpkin ball will be easier for the younger children to move. Younger children can also practice skills with the pumpkin ball such as rolling, pushing, and kicking the ball. If your school only has one cage ball, this can be done in a shuttle formation.

TEACHING HINTS

Watch for children, especially younger ones, who have a difficult time staying out of the pumpkin-ball area. Also watch for those students who "hog" the playground balls. Tell them they must share the balls.

Stress that the students use correct throwing form when they are playing the game.

Ghosts and Goblins

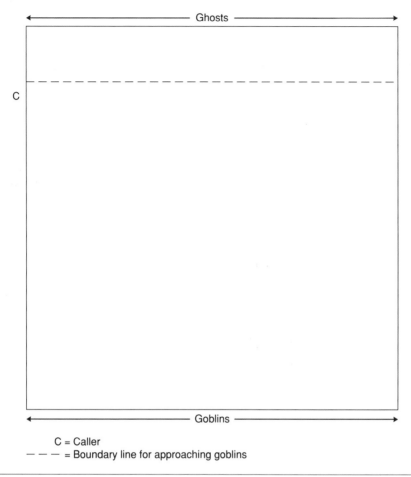

C = Caller
− − − = Boundary line for approaching goblins

Figure 2.7 Ghosts and goblins.

QUICK DESCRIPTION

A chasing and fleeing game (Figure 2.7)

APPROPRIATE GRADES

K-3

ACTIVITY GOALS

To demonstrate bodily control and knowledge of game and safety rules in a game situation

SPACE REQUIRED

Large outside area or gymnasium

KEY SKILLS

Running, chasing, fleeing, dodging, tagging safely, and developing honesty and good sportsmanship

EQUIPMENT AND PREPARATION

Mark off a large playing area with two end lines. Traffic cones may be used.

ACTIVITY PROCEDURE

Divide the class, as evenly as possible, into two groups. One group will be the "ghosts" and the other will be the "goblins." Line up the goblins at one end of the playing area. Then line up the ghosts at the other end and have them turn around so they are facing away from the goblins. Emphasize that there must be no peeking. To begin the game, a caller gives the goblins a hand signal. This is their cue to start sneaking up very quietly on the ghosts. When they get close to the ghosts the caller says, "The goblins are coming!" This is the signal for the ghosts to turn around and try to catch the goblins before they get back to their starting position. The ghosts keep count of the number of goblins they tag. Then both groups return to their original starting positions and the game is repeated with the roles reversed.

SAFETY CONSIDERATIONS

Emphasize that the students tag lightly. They should not push people or grab clothing.

When playing outdoors, grass is preferable to blacktop to prevent scrapes if someone does fall down.

Keep the end lines a safe distance from walls or fences so the students don't run into them. Say, "The ghosts/goblins are coming," before the students reach the ghosts or goblins to prevent collisions when they turn around quickly.

ADAPTATION SUGGESTIONS

Other locomotor skills, such as galloping and skipping, can be used in the chasing part of the game.

The size of the playing area can be adapted for each class.

TEACHING HINTS

Some students will try to peek, either over their shoulder or between their legs. This peeking usually upsets the group that is sneaking up. Have the student that continues to peek sit out for one game.

If some students are afraid to sneak up close to the other team, mark a line that they must sneak up to.

Black Cat Stretches

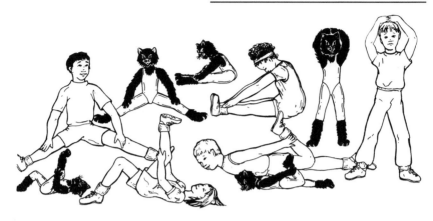

Figure 2.8 Black cat stretches.

QUICK DESCRIPTION

Flexibility exercises that can be used as a warm-up or cool-down for any of the Halloween activities (Figure 2.8)

APPROPRIATE GRADES

K-6

ACTIVITY GOALS

To perform the static stretching exercises correctly and to develop flexibility

SPACE REQUIRED

Gymnasium or large classroom

KEY SKILLS

Learning static stretching exercises

EQUIPMENT AND PREPARATION

Select some flexibility exercises to use. Remember to include all the large muscle groups. You will need **a record or cassette player** and **a slow, relaxing piece of music**.

ACTIVITY PROCEDURE

Ask students to describe how a cat moves when it wakes up from a nap. Tell them that they are going to move in a slow, relaxed, catlike manner when they perform the flexibility exercises. Explain the correct way to perform each exercise and tell them which muscles are being stretched. Students should hold each stretch for 5 to 30 seconds, depending on their ability. Play the music softly in the background while the students perform the exercises.

SAFETY CONSIDERATIONS

During each flexibility exercise, students should gradually increase the stretch to the point of discomfort, but not to the point of pain. They should be able to hold the stretched position comfortably. There is no bouncing in static stretching.

ADAPTATION SUGGESTIONS

Choose flexibility exercises for all the major muscle groups. Emphasize those groups on which the lesson is concentrated.

TEACHING HINTS

Walk among the students and correct their form as needed. Stress the importance of correct form.

Shaky Skeleton Dance

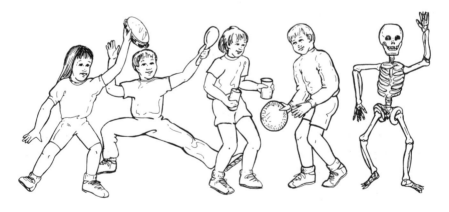

Figure 2.9   Shaky skeleton dance.

QUICK DESCRIPTION
Fundamental rhythms and creative dance activity (Figure 2.9)

APPROPRIATE GRADES
K-3

ACTIVITY GOALS
To perform locomotor and nonlocomotor skills with and without a rhythm instrument to the beat of the music, and to respond creatively to the music

SPACE REQUIRED
Gymnasium or large classroom

KEY SKILLS
Developing a sense of rhythm, performing various locomotor and nonlocomotor skills to music, manipulating a rhythm instrument to the beat of the music, and developing creativity

EQUIPMENT AND PREPARATION
You will need **a record or cassette player** and **a lively piece of music** to which the children will respond well. "Shake, Rattle, and Roll" is a good one (Bill Haley and the Comets, Decca Records). Ask the music teacher in your school if you can borrow **some rhythm instruments** that make a sound when shaken. Ideally, you should have one instrument for each student. If you don't have enough instruments for each student, make some by putting stones or beans in a can or box with a lid, or between two paper plates that are stapled together. Tape the lid closed to prevent stones or beans from escaping. You will also need **a picture of the muscular system—** ideally, one that shows all the major systems of the body—and **a picture of the skeletal system**.

ACTIVITY PROCEDURE
Tell the students that you are turning them into skeletons. Show them the pictures of the body systems and talk about each one for a few minutes. Tell them that the only system they will be able to use today is the skeletal system, which consists of bones. When they move, they must pretend that they are made only of bones.

1. Without music, ask the students to walk, run, gallop, skip, jump, slide, and hop while pretending they are skeletons.

2. Without music, have them shake various body parts, such as the hands, legs, head, elbows, shoulders, and entire body.

3. Have them sit down and listen to the music. Then have them perform the same skills to music.

4. Pass out the rhythm instruments and let the students practice shaking them in various stationary positions, such as standing, sitting, kneeling, and lying down. Then have them shake the instruments while performing locomotor skills (walking, running, hopping, jumping, galloping, skipping, and sliding).

5. Have the students perform the stationary shaking and locomotor skills while shaking the rhythm instruments to the music.

6. Finally, play the music and allow the students to create their own shaky skeleton dance using the previously learned skills.

Students can perform their dances for each other.

SAFETY CONSIDERATIONS

Emphasize the importance of moving safely in personal and general space. When using the instruments, make sure the students have enough room to avoid accidentally hitting each other.

ADAPTATION SUGGESTIONS

Use skills the students have already mastered. These skills will vary with different grade levels and with students with disabilities.

TEACHING HINTS

When you give the instructions, tell the students to place their rhythm instruments on the floor so they can't make noise with them.

If some students purposely fall down too much during the activities, ask them to please stay on their feet.

Chapter 3

NOVEMBER

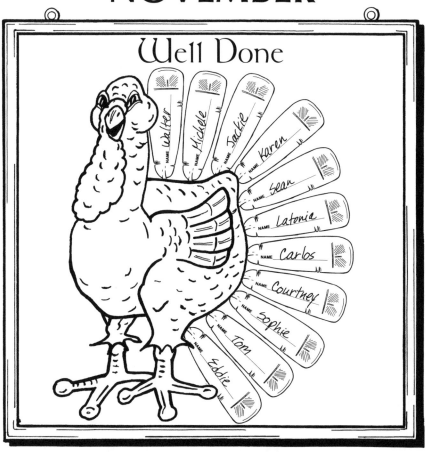

THANKSGIVING

"Well-Done" Turkey Trot

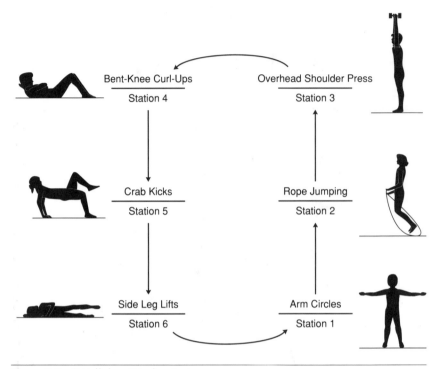

Figure 3.1 "Well-done" turkey trot.

QUICK DESCRIPTION

Physical fitness exercise circuit training course (Figure 3.1)

APPROPRIATE GRADES

K-6

ACTIVITY GOALS

To improve physical fitness levels, especially muscular strength and endurance and cardiovascular endurance, by motivating students to put more effort into the physical fitness exercises

SPACE REQUIRED

Gymnasium, track, or large outside area

KEY SKILLS

The November circuit training course emphasizes the following skills:

- Arm and shoulder girdle strength and endurance (arm circles, overhead shoulder press with hand weights, crab kicks)

- General body conditioning (rope jumping)
- Abdominal strength and endurance (bent-knee curl-ups)
- Leg strength and endurance (crab kicks, side leg lifts)
- Cardiovascular endurance (jogging)

EQUIPMENT AND PREPARATION

Start this circuit training course at the beginning of November. For the sample circuit training course, construct **7 signs**, one for each of the six exercise stations, and one that says "Well Done." The station signs should be "Arm Circles," "Rope Jumping," "Overhead Shoulder Press," "Bent-Knee Curl-Ups," "Crab Kicks," and "Side Leg Lifts." Using construction paper, make **1 large turkey body** and enough **paper feathers** (Figure A.6 in the appendix) for each of your students. Make the body of the turkey large enough to accommodate the number of feathers that will be added to it.

NOTE: This is an excellent art project for a cooperating classroom or art teacher. One large turkey, or several smaller turkeys for each class, can be created. Every student can make his or her own feather. Feathers should be of different colors and each should have the student's name printed on it.

Attach the turkey body (or numerous turkey bodies) to a wall or bulletin board where everyone can see it, and place the "Well Done" sign above the turkey. Set up the exercise stations. You will need **6 traffic cones, 4 jump ropes**, and **4 or 5 pairs of 1- to 3-pound hand weights**.

Build excitement and interest by telling the students that they are going to help create the biggest and most beautiful turkey by exercising. Put up signs around the school that say "Help Build the Largest Turkey! Coming Soon in Physical Education Classes."

ACTIVITY PROCEDURE

Review the activity procedures for circuit training courses on page xii. Allow 15 to 20 seconds for each station.

Students earn a turkey feather with their name on it to add to the turkey body the first time they correctly complete the course. They receive a brightly colored check (made with marker or crayon) on their feather every time they complete the course after that.

SAFETY CONSIDERATIONS

Emphasize correct form while performing the exercises. Tell the students to place the hand weights away from the jogging area when they are finished using them.

ADAPTATION SUGGESTIONS

For the younger students, the jog between stations can either be omitted or the circumference of the circuit can be reduced. Other locomotor or nonlocomotor activities, such as animal walks, skipping, and galloping, can be substituted for some of the exercises.

Give children with disabilities appropriate adapted movement challenges.

TEACHING HINTS

Choose exercises with which the children are already familiar. You can use cans of food in place of hand weights.

Tricky Turkey
and Sailing to Plymouth Rock

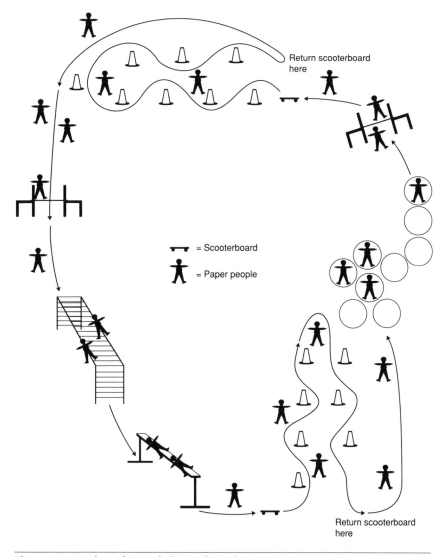

Return scooterboard here

= Scooterboard

= Paper people

Return scooterboard here

Figure 3.2 Tricky turkey and Plymouth Rock.

QUICK DESCRIPTION

Obstacle course (Figure 3.2)

APPROPRIATE GRADES

K-6

ACTIVITY GOALS

To complete the skills in the obstacle course correctly while touching a minimum number of obstacles

SPACE REQUIRED

Gymnasium

KEY SKILLS

Demonstrating bodily control while performing the entire obstacle course; using perceptual motor skills; propelling self with hands only while lying in a prone position on the scooterboard and with feet only while sitting on the scooterboard; performing various forms of locomotion on the balance beam; crab-walking on the horizontal ladder; performing various forms of locomotion through the Hula Hoops or tires; and climbing over and crawling under various obstacles

EQUIPMENT AND PREPARATION

Reproduce about **30 paper people shapes** (Figure A.7a in the appendix) and enough **"Tricky Turkey" certificates** (Figure A.7b in the appendix) **or "I Landed on Plymouth Rock" certificates** (Figure A.7c in the appendix) for everyone in your class. Assemble the obstacle course. If you are doing the "Tricky Turkey" course, attach the paper people in various places along the course. There is nothing to attach for the "Plymouth Rock" course. You will need **2 scooterboards, 15 traffic cones, 1 low balance beam, 10 Hula Hoops or tires, 4 chairs, 2 sticks** about 6 yards long, **1 horizontal ladder**, and enough **mats** to place around equipment such as the balance beam and horizontal ladder.

To motivate students, put up signs around the school about a week before the event that say "Will You Be Caught for Thanksgiving Dinner?" "Are You a Tricky Turkey or Turkey Dinner?" or "Will You Land on Plymouth Rock?"

ACTIVITY PROCEDURE

Review the activity procedures for obstacle courses on page xiii. Explain the obstacle course to the class. If the students touch a paper person it means the students have been caught for Thanksgiving dinner. If they make it through the course without touching any paper people, it means they have been tricky turkeys and have escaped successfully. They then receive a "Tricky Turkey" certificate. If the students pretend to be pilgrims and touch five or fewer obstacles, it means they have landed on Plymouth Rock, and they receive an "I Landed on Plymouth Rock" certificate.

These are the activities included in the sample course:

• Sitting on a scooterboard and maneuvering in and out of the cones using the feet only while holding the scooterboard with the hands

- Jumping on two feet from hoop to hoop without touching the hoops
- Crawling under the low stick
- Lying on scooterboard in a prone (face down) position and maneuvering in and out of cones using the arms only
- Climbing over the high stick
- Performing the crab walk across the horizontal ladder
- Walking on the balance beam

SAFETY CONSIDERATIONS

Emphasize that students begin on the signal and stop when they complete the course. Make sure you place enough mats around the balance beam, horizontal ladder, and any other areas where they are necessary.

ADAPTATION SUGGESTIONS

Vary the activities according to skill level. For example, for younger children, lower the stick that they climb over. To make the course more challenging, move the cones for the scooterboard activity closer together. Adapt activities appropriately for children with physical disabilities.

TEACHING HINTS

Choose activities with which the children are familiar.

At the end of class, ask the students if their partners performed the skills correctly and if they touched any of the paper people or obstacles.

Thanksgiving Skills Stations

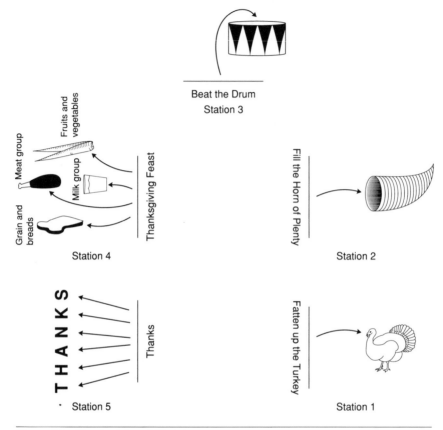

Figure 3.3 Thanksgiving skill stations.

QUICK DESCRIPTION
Throwing skills stations (Figure 3.3)

APPROPRIATE GRADES
K-6

ACTIVITY GOALS
To improve form and accuracy while performing the underhand and overhand throw

SPACE REQUIRED
Gymnasium

KEY SKILLS

Underhand and overhand throwing

EQUIPMENT AND PREPARATION

Construct **5 signs**, one for each of the stations: "Fatten up the Turkey," "Fill the Horn of Plenty," "Beat the Drum," "Thanksgiving Feast," and "Thanks." Also make the following targets: **a picture of a turkey, a picture of a horn of plenty, a picture of an Indian drum, pictures of foods from the different food groups** (these can be cut out of magazines), and **the letters that spell the word "Thanks"** cut from construction paper.

Attach the signs and pictures to the wall where each station will be. Using **masking tape**, mark lines on the floor that the students must stand behind when they throw. You will also need **5 traffic cones** (one for each station) to designate where the stations are located, and **10 beanbags** (two for each station).

ACTIVITY PROCEDURE

Review the activity procedures for skills stations on page xiv. Explain each station to the class.

Station Description

- Fatten Up the Turkey—Students pretend that the beanbags are food and throw them at the turkey's mouth.
- Fill the Horn of Plenty—Students pretend the beanbags are fruit and throw them at the opening of the Horn of Plenty.
- Beat the Indian Drum—Students hit (beat) the head of the drum with the beanbags.
- Thanksgiving Feast—Students must call out which picture of the different food groups they are trying to hit before they throw the beanbags.
- Thanks—Students must hit the letters in correct spelling order. Students begin with the "T." If they hit it, they aim for the "H" with the second beanbag. If they hit the "H," the students aim for the "A" on their next turn. If the "H" is missed, then the "H" will be aimed for on the next turn.

SAFETY CONSIDERATIONS

Make sure that the students who are waiting aren't too close to the student who is throwing or in the target area.

ADAPTATION SUGGESTIONS

The students can first practice the underhand and overhand throws. Lower or raise the targets according to the ages of the students. Also, shorten or lengthen the distance from the throwing line to the target according to skill level. Adjust the skills for children with disabilities.

TEACHING HINTS

Teach students correct throwing form before they practice at the stations.

Students can draw the pictures for you or you can purchase Thanksgiving picture decorations at any card shop.

Thankful Turkey Tag

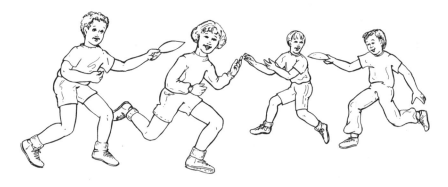

Figure 3.4   Thankful turkey tag.

QUICK DESCRIPTION

A chasing and fleeing game (Figure 3.4)

APPROPRIATE GRADES

K-6

ACTIVITY GOALS

To demonstrate bodily control and knowledge of game and safety rules in a game situation

SPACE REQUIRED

Gymnasium or outside area with marked boundaries

KEY SKILLS

Running, chasing, fleeing, dodging, and tagging safely; and developing honesty and good sportsmanship

EQUIPMENT AND PREPARATION

You will need a **few large pieces of paper** with a class's name printed on each of them, **some crayons or markers**, and **3 or 4 real or paper feathers** (Figure A.6 in the appendix), depending on the number of children who will be "it." You may need **some traffic cones** to mark the boundaries.

ACTIVITY PROCEDURE

Students designated as "it" are the turkeys. Each turkey carries a feather with which to tag the other players.

Well-defined boundaries are needed whether the game is played inside or outside. Players who go outside the boundaries are considered tagged. Begin the game by saying "Gobble, gobble." This is the signal for the turkeys to try to tag as many of the other players as they can. When players are tagged, they must write something for which they are thankful and their names on the large sheets of paper. After doing this, players rejoin the game.

SAFETY CONSIDERATIONS

Emphasize the correct way to tag someone with the feather. Students should tag on the arms, legs, back, or chest, and not the head or face. They should not push or grab clothing when they are trying to tag someone. Also emphasize that they watch where they are running at all times to avoid collisions. Clear the playing area of dangerous objects and hazards, such as chairs, tables, and other equipment. Keep the boundaries away from walls to avoid accidents.

ADAPTATION SUGGESTIONS

Because younger children will tire more quickly, having fewer turkeys might be better. That way they will not be chased so much. If you provide more turkeys for older children, the extra running will give them more aerobic exercise. Older children can keep score by counting the number of times they are tagged. Those tagged the fewest times are the winners.

TEACHING HINTS

Choose one to four students to be "it." Larger classes will need more turkeys so that all the children will have an opportunity to be chased. This also gives more children a chance to be "it."

Change taggers frequently so that many children have the opportunity to be "it."

Watch for children who like to chase only their friends. If you have students who don't like to participate, choose them to be the taggers or add more taggers.

At the end of the game, gather the class in front of the papers where the students have listed the things for which they are thankful. Have the class read them. At this time, students who never got tagged may write something for which they are thankful on the paper. Each class's list can be taped to the wall for everyone to see.

Indian Dance

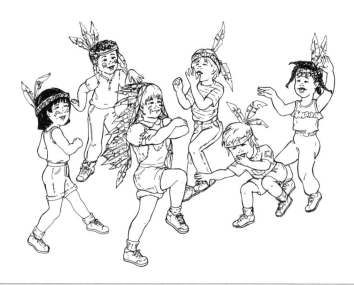

Figure 3.5   Indian dance.

QUICK DESCRIPTION

Fundamental rhythms and creative dance activity (Figure 3.5)

APPROPRIATE GRADES

K-3

ACTIVITY GOALS

To perform locomotor and nonlocomotor skills to the beat of a drum and to respond creatively to the drumbeat using the same skills

SPACE REQUIRED

Gymnasium or large classroom

KEY SKILLS

Developing a sense of rhythm, performing various locomotor and nonlocomotor skills to a drumbeat, and responding creatively to a drumbeat

EQUIPMENT AND PREPARATION

Students can make their own Indian headbands with feathers (Figure A.6 in the appendix) out of construction paper to wear when they perform their creative Indian dances.

NOTE: This is an excellent art project for a cooperating classroom teacher or art teacher.

Each student will need **one 1- to 2-inch-wide strip of construction paper** long enough to fit around the head like a sweatband. The students should then cut out about **8 paper feathers** of different colors and decorate them with **crayons, markers, or paint**. Then they can paste or otherwise attach the feathers to each headband. The students can bring the feathered headbands to physical education class on the day they will perform their creative Indian dances.

You will also need **a drum or tom-tom**.

ACTIVITY PROCEDURE

Students should be familiar with beat, tempo, measure, accent, intensity, and phrase. Review and define these terms. Explain to the students that they will be using these characteristics of music when they move to the drumbeat. Begin by having students tap different parts of their bodies with their hands to the drumbeat. Then they can perform nonlocomotor skills such as shaking, swaying, twisting, turning, bending, stretching, bouncing, raising, and lowering to the beat of the drum.

Next they can perform locomotor skills such as walking, running, galloping, hopping, skipping, leaping, and sliding. Beat the drum at different tempos (speeds) and intensities (light or heavy), and place accents on different beats. Instruct the students to move in different directions, in different patterns, at different levels, and with different body parts leading. Once the students are performing the skills to the drumbeat well, explain that they will create their own Thanksgiving Indian dances using the skills they have been practicing. Tell them that they can decide which skills to perform and how to move. Everyone's dance will be different. For the creative Indian dance, beat the drum in a variety of rhythms so the students can respond creatively in many ways. Students can wear their Indian head-bands when they perform their creative dances. Half the class can watch the other half perform to see all the different ideas. You could also invite the art and classroom teachers to watch.

SAFETY CONSIDERATIONS

Emphasize the importance of moving safely in personal and general space.

ADAPTATION SUGGESTIONS

Use skills that the students have mastered. These skills will vary with the different grade levels and with children with disabilities.

TEACHING HINTS

When creating their own Indian dances, some students may copy the movements of others. Encourage them to "do their own thing." There are usually a few students who will just run around no matter how you beat the drum. Stop these students and let them observe for a few minutes to get the feel of what the class is doing. Point out students who are performing correctly. Please teach your students to understand and respect Native American culture when they create their Thanksgiving Indian dances.

Turkey in the Straw

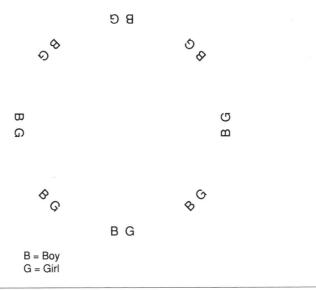

Figure 3.6 "Turkey in the Straw" dance.

QUICK DESCRIPTION
Folk dance (Figure 3.6)

APPROPRIATE GRADES
K-6

ACTIVITY GOALS
To perform the dance "Turkey in the Straw" correctly and to improve the ability to work cooperatively in a group

SPACE REQUIRED
Gymnasium or large classroom

KEY SKILLS
Walking or sliding and skipping to music in a circle and with a partner.

EQUIPMENT AND PREPARATION
You will need **a record or cassette player** and **a recording of "Turkey in the Straw."** You should be able to find it at the public library.

ACTIVITY PROCEDURE
Pair off boys and girls together. Arrange the couples in a single circle. Couples should face the center of the circle with the girl to the right of the

boy. Have everyone join hands. Young children (K-3) don't have to be paired off boy/girl. They usually don't care who their partner is as long as they are dancing.

The dance is performed in 4/4 time.

MEASURES

1-2   Beginning with the left foot, students take seven walking steps or slides to the left (they hold to the count of eight and prepare to change directions).

3-4   Beginning with the right foot, students take seven walking steps or slides to the right (they hold to the count of eight).

5   Beginning with the left foot, students walk two steps to the center of the circle (weight should be on both feet) and clap three times.

6   Beginning with the right foot, students walk two steps backward to the start (weight should be on both feet) and clap three times.

7-8   Students hook their right elbows with their partners' and turn in place using a walking or skipping step. The dance continues by repeating Measures 1 through 8. To make the dance a mixer (changing partners) and more challenging for older students, have the boys leave their present partners during Measure 8 and walk or skip in a counterclockwise direction to meet new partners. Have the girls step in place during this measure. Then the dance continues by repeating Measures 1 through 8.

SAFETY CONSIDERATIONS

Students get very excited when there is lively music. Some students, especially younger ones, like to fall down purposely when the class is in a circle with hands joined or when performing the elbow swing. Emphasize that this is unacceptable. If someone falls down accidentally, the class should know that they are to stop the dance.

ADAPTATION SUGGESTIONS

Younger students can use walking steps until they are ready to slide and skip. Older students should be able to perform the dance as a mixer in boy/girl couples.

TEACHING HINTS

Have the students clap to the beat of the music before learning the steps so they can become familiar with it. Students should know how to slide and skip before learning the dance.

Chapter 4

DECEMBER/JANUARY

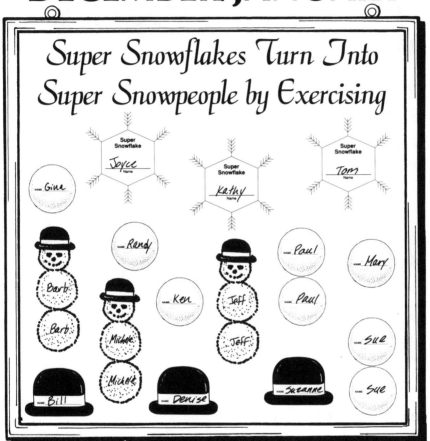

Super Snowflakes Turn Into Super Snowpeople by Exercising

WINTER, CHRISTMAS, HANUKKAH

Super Snowflakes Turn Into Super Snowpeople by Exercising

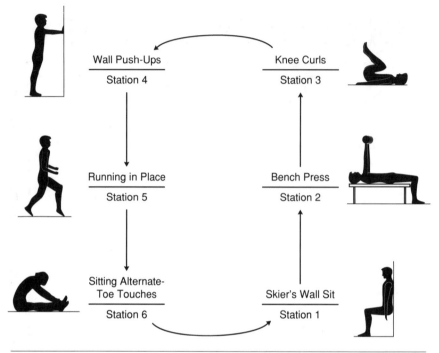

Figure 4.1 Super snowflakes turn into super snowpeople by exercising.

QUICK DESCRIPTION

Physical fitness exercise circuit training course (Figure 4.1)

APPROPRIATE GRADES

K-6

ACTIVITY GOALS

To improve physical fitness levels, especially muscular strength and endurance and cardiovascular endurance, by motivating the students to put more effort into the physical fitness exercises

SPACE REQUIRED

Gymnasium, track, or large outside area

KEY SKILLS

The winter circuit training course emphasizes the following skills:

- Leg strength (skier's wall sit)
- Arm and shoulder girdle strength and endurance (bench press with hand weights, wall push-ups)
- Abdominal strength and endurance (knee curls)
- General body conditioning (running in place)
- Trunk strength (sitting alternate-toe touches)
- Cardiovascular endurance (jogging, aerobic dancing, or paper-plate or carpet-square skating)

EQUIPMENT AND PREPARATION

Start this circuit training course at the beginning of December. For the sample circuit training course, construct **7 signs**, one for each of the exercise stations and one that says "Super Snowflakes Turn Into Super Snowpeople by Exercising." The station signs should be "Skier's Wall Sit," "Bench Press," "Knee Curls," "Wall Push-Ups," "Running in Place," and "Sitting Alternate-Toe Touches." Reproduce enough **paper "super snowflakes" certificates** (Figure A.8a in the appendix), **paper snowballs** (Figure A.8b in the appendix), and **paper top hats** (Figure A.8c in the appendix) for everyone in your class.

Attach the "Super Snowflakes Turn Into Super Snowpeople by Exercising" sign to a wall or bulletin board where everyone can see it, and set up the exercise stations. You will need **6 traffic cones** and **4 or 5 pairs of 1- to 3-pound hand weights**.

Optional equipment: Seasonal records or cassettes, a record or cassette player, and 2 paper plates or carpet squares for each student.

Build excitement and interest by putting up signs around the school about a week before the event that say "You Can Turn a Snowflake Into a Snowball, and a Snowball Into a Snowperson in Physical Education Class!" or "How Many Snowpeople Can You Build by Exercising?"

ACTIVITY PROCEDURE

Review the activity procedures for circuit training courses on page xii. Allow 15 to 20 seconds for each station.

Students earn a super snowflake the first time they correctly complete the course, a snowball the second, third, and fourth times, and a top hat the fifth time, thus completing the snowperson. Students can draw faces on their snowpeople in their free time.

Repeat this award procedure depending on the number of times students complete the course.

SAFETY CONSIDERATIONS

Emphasize that students use correct form while they perform the exercises. Tell the children to watch out for students who lose their "skates" and go back after them. Instruct students to place the hand weights away from the jogging area when they are finished using them.

ADAPTATION SUGGESTIONS

Instead of jogging, students can "skate" on paper plates or carpet squares. When students are using the paper plates or carpet squares to "skate," make the circumference of the lap area smaller than if they were jogging. "Skating" is more difficult than jogging and takes more time. You can substitute teacher- or student-led aerobic dancing to seasonal music for the jogging or skating. You can alternate days of jogging, "skating," and aerobic dancing.

TEACHING HINTS

Choose exercises and aerobic dance steps with which the children are familiar.

You can substitute cans of food for hand weights.

Winter Wonderful Land

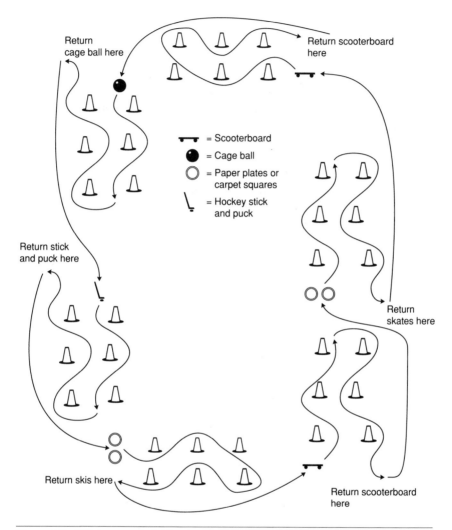

Return cage ball here

Return scooterboard here

= Scooterboard

= Cage ball

= Paper plates or carpet squares

= Hockey stick and puck

Return stick and puck here

Return skates here

Return skis here

Return scooterboard here

Figure 4.2 Winter wonderful land.

QUICK DESCRIPTION

Obstacle course (Figure 4.2)

APPROPRIATE GRADES

K-6

ACTIVITY GOALS

To complete the skills in the obstacle course correctly while touching a minimum number of obstacles

SPACE REQUIRED

Gymnasium

KEY SKILLS

Demonstrating bodily control while performing the entire obstacle course; using perceptual motor skills; "skiing" forward and "skating" backward on carpet squares or paper plates; maneuvering scooterboards through obstacles while lying in a prone position and also while sitting on them; maneuvering a cage ball through obstacles; and maneuvering a hockey puck with a hockey stick through obstacles

EQUIPMENT AND PREPARATION

Reproduce enough **"I Was Winter Wonderful" certificates** (Figure A.9 in the appendix) for everyone in your class. Assemble the obstacle course. You will need **5 pairs of carpet squares or paper plates, 4 scooterboards, 2 floor hockey sticks, 2 hockey pucks, 1 cage ball, 36 traffic cones** or other type of marker, and **6 folding tumbling mats.**

Motivate students by putting up signs the week before the course is run that say "Take a Trip Through the Land of Snow and Ice" or "Pretend You Are in the Winter Olympics."

ACTIVITY PROCEDURE

Review the activity procedures for obstacle courses on page xiii. Explain the obstacle course. Students who complete the course correctly and touch five or fewer cones, receive an "I Was Winter Wonderful" certificate. The following activities are included in the sample course:

- *Tobogganing*—Students sit on scooterboards and move through obstacles.
- *Skating*—Students "skate" backwards on carpet squares or paper plates through obstacles.
- *Sledding*—Students lie prone (face down) on scooterboards and move through obstacles.
- *Snowman Building*—Students roll a cage ball through obstacles.
- *Ice Hockey*—Students hit a hockey puck through obstacles with a hockey stick.
- *Skiing*—Students "ski" forward on carpet squares or paper plates.

SAFETY CONSIDERATIONS

Emphasize that students start on the signal and stop when they complete the course.

ADAPTATION SUGGESTIONS

Increase or decrease the distances in which each skill must be performed according to the skill level of the students. You can also adjust the number of obstacles you allow them to touch.

TEACHING HINTS

Tell the students to return the scooterboard, cage ball, "skates" to the starting position for the next person.

Winter and Holiday Skills Stations

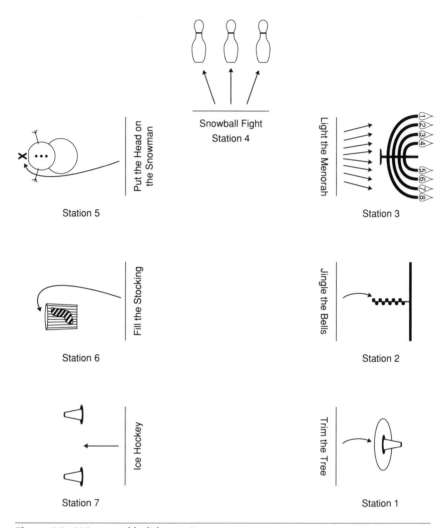

Figure 4.3 Winter and holiday stations.

QUICK DESCRIPTION

Ball-handling and striking skills stations (Figure 4.3)

APPROPRIATE GRADES

K-6

ACTIVITY GOALS

To improve form and accuracy while performing the following ball-handling and striking skills: rolling, underhand throwing, overhand throwing, overhead volleying, and striking with a racket and hockey stick

SPACE REQUIRED

Gymnasium

KEY SKILLS

Rolling, underhand throwing, overhand throwing, striking with a racket and hockey stick, and the overhead volley

EQUIPMENT AND PREPARATION

Prepare the following seven stations:

• *Trim the Tree*—Construct **a sign** that says "Trim the Tree." Cover **a large traffic cone** with **green paper** to make a Christmas tree. You will also need **2 hoops or rings**.

• *Jingle the Bells*—Construct **a sign** that says "Jingle the Bells." Tie **some jingle bells** on **a piece of string** and suspend them from **a bar**. You will also need **2 beanbags or small balls**.

• *Light the Menorah*—Construct **a sign** that says "Light the Menorah." Make from **construction paper** a Menorah (an eight-branched candelabrum with an extra branch called the "Shammas," which is used to light the other eight lights). Make **8 paper candles** and number them 1 through 8. You will also need **8 beanbags**.

• *Snowball Fight*—Construct **a sign** that says "Snowball Fight." You will need **2 fleece, yarn, or sponge balls** or **2 old rolled-up socks**, and **2 plastic bowling pins** or other targets.

• *Put the Head on the Snowman*—Construct **a sign** that says "Put the Head on the Snowman." Make **2 large circles** using **white paper** to resemble a snowman's body. You will also need **a volleyball**.

• *Fill the Stocking*—Construct **a sign** that says "Fill the Stocking." Make **a picture of a Christmas stocking** and attach it to **a trash barrel**. You will also need **1 racket or paddle** and **1 ball**.

• *Ice Hockey*—Construct **a sign** that says "Ice Hockey." You will also need **2 traffic cones, 1 hockey stick**, and **1 hockey puck**.

Set up the stations in the gym and put the corresponding signs on the wall. Mark lines on the floor with **masking tape** behind which the students must stand when taking their turns.

ACTIVITY PROCEDURE

Review the activity procedures for skills stations on page xiv. Explain each station to the class.

Station Description

• *Trim the Tree*—Students throw the hoops or rings at the tree, trying to ring the cone.

- *Jingle the Bells*—Students jingle the bells by throwing the balls or beanbags at them.

- *Light the Menorah*—Students hit the flames of the candles in numerical order with the beanbags.

- *Snowball Fight*—Students hit the bowling pins or other targets with the balls or socks.

- *Put the Head on the Snowman*—Using an overhead volley or overhead throw, students hit the spot where the snowman's head should be.

- *Fill the Stocking*—Students hit the ball into the barrel using a racket or paddle.

- *Ice Hockey*—Students hit the puck into the goal with the hockey stick.

SAFETY CONSIDERATIONS

Tell students to stand away from the person who is taking a turn so they don't get hit accidentally. This is especially important at the hockey and racket stations.

ADAPTATION SUGGESTIONS

Younger students can progress from rolling at the targets to throwing. Lower the targets for rolling. Shorten or lengthen the distance from the restraining line to the target depending on skill level. You may not want to use all seven stations at once. Select a few at a time.

TEACHING HINTS

Teach the skills to the students before they practice at the stations.

Indoor Snowballs

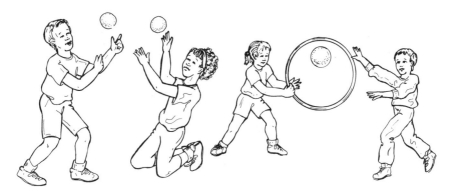

Figure 4.4 Indoor snowballs.

QUICK DESCRIPTION
Ball-handling skills (Figure 4.4)

APPROPRIATE GRADES
K-3

ACTIVITY GOALS
To improve skill level in tossing to oneself, catching, underhand throwing, overhand throwing, and striking

SPACE REQUIRED
Gymnasium

KEY SKILLS
Tossing to oneself, catching, underhand throwing, overhand throwing, and striking

EQUIPMENT AND PREPARATION
You will need **1 "snowball" for each child**. The snowballs can be fleece or yarn balls or rolled-up socks. You will also need **1 Hula Hoop for every two children**.

ACTIVITY PROCEDURE
Students should practice the following activities with both their right and left hands, where appropriate.

Individual Activities

Tossing and Catching

- Tossing and catching, gradually increasing the height of the toss
- Tossing, clapping hands, and catching
- Tossing, turning around, and catching
- Tossing underneath the right leg and catching and tossing underneath the left leg and catching
- Tossing from the right hand to the left hand and from the left hand to the right hand
- Tossing and catching at different levels

Striking

- Tossing the snowball and striking it upward from underneath with an open hand
- Tossing the snowball and striking it forward with an open hand overhead, as in volleyball
- Tossing the snowball and striking it forward with an open hand out to the side, like a tennis forehand drive
- Striking the snowball with different body parts

Partner Activities

- Rolling the snowball to a partner
- Throwing underhand to a partner
- Throwing overhand to a partner
- Tossing upward and striking the snowball underhand to a partner
- Tossing upward and striking the snowball overhand to a partner
- Tossing upward and striking the snowball with the hand out to the side
- Throwing to a partner from different levels and in different body positions
- A third student holds a Hula Hoop for the snowball to go through while the partners throw and catch; they can rotate positions so that each one gets to hold the hoop
- Partners throwing two snowballs at the same time
- Partners volleying the snowballs as in volleyball

SAFETY CONSIDERATIONS

Students should have enough space to avoid collisions. Tell them to spread out and be aware of other students.

ADAPTATION SUGGESTIONS

Allow students to progress at their own speed. You can give more challenging skills to those students who are ready.

TEACHING HINTS

If you are using socks, ask the students to bring old white socks to school to use for the snowballs.

Emphasize correct form when students are performing the skills. Also stress that they throw the ball so that they or their partners can catch it easily. They should not throw hard and wild, but control the ball.

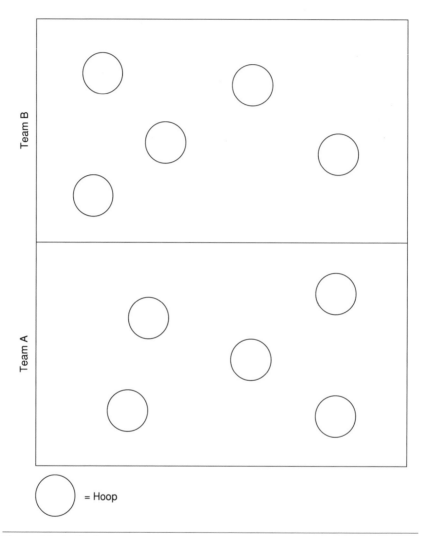

Team B

Team A

◯ = Hoop

Figure 4.5 In the freezer.

QUICK DESCRIPTION

A throwing-for-accuracy team game (Figure 4.5)

APPROPRIATE GRADES

K-6

ACTIVITY GOALS

To use the skills of throwing for accuracy and blocking in a game situation

SPACE REQUIRED

An area the size of a volleyball court with a center dividing line

KEY SKILLS

Throwing for accuracy, blocking, participating cooperatively in a team game, obeying the rules of a game, and demonstrating knowledge of safety rules while playing a game

EQUIPMENT AND PREPARATION

You will need **20 or more fleece, yarn, or sponge balls, or rolled-up socks** (ideally one per player), **8 to 10 targets** (for example, boxes, trash cans, hoops, or any type of container that the balls can be thrown into), and **traffic cones** (if you need to mark off the playing area).

ACTIVITY PROCEDURE

Divide the class, as evenly as possible, into two teams. Have each team scatter on one half of the playing area with an equal number of snowballs. Identically position an equal number of "freezers" (targets) on each team's side. When you give the signal, players throw as many of the snowballs into the freezers on the opposite side as they can. Players cannot cross the center dividing line nor can they reach over the dividing line to get snowballs. Players can prevent snowballs from entering the freezers by catching or striking them. They can stand behind or to the side of the freezers, but they cannot stand directly in front of them, straddle them, or sit on them. Once a snowball enters a freezer, it remains there until the end of the game. The team that throws the most snowballs into the freezers wins. Repeat the game as desired.

SAFETY CONSIDERATIONS

Stress that the students watch out for others as they block and retrieve balls.

ADAPTATION SUGGESTIONS

Adjust the distance the freezers are placed from the center dividing line according to skill level.

TEACHING HINTS

If you are using socks for the snowballs, ask students to bring old, clean, white socks to school. They will probably bring more than enough.

Watch for students who don't follow the rules. For example, some students may reach over the dividing line to get a snowball or stand in front of the freezers. If they continue to break the rules, have them sit out for a while.

Muscletoe

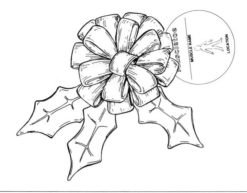

Figure 4.6 Muscletoe.

QUICK DESCRIPTION

Holiday muscle-name learning game that uses decorations resembling mistletoe (Figure 4.6)

APPROPRIATE GRADES

K-6

ACTIVITY GOALS

To name and locate muscles on the body by making holiday decorations

SPACE REQUIRED

A section of the gymnasium or classroom

KEY SKILLS

Demonstrating knowledge of major muscle groups and their locations

EQUIPMENT AND PREPARATION

To make each "muscletoe" decoration you will need some type of **artificial holiday greenery**, for example, a package of green garland cut into 6-inch pieces. You will also need **ribbon** to make bows for the muscletoe, and **twist ties**. Reproduce one **muscletoe name and location card** (Figure A.10 in the appendix) for each muscletoe you make. You will also need **markers**.

ACTIVITY PROCEDURE

Making muscletoe is very easy. Take a piece of garland and fold it in half to make it look fuller. Secure it with a twist tie. Tie on the ribbon and make a bow. Write the name of a muscle and check off its location on the muscle card. Then attach the muscle card to the twist tie. Students can choose which muscle name they want on their muscletoe. Try to have all of the major muscle groups written on the muscletoe used to decorate the school.

Students can make the muscletoe to decorate the school or to give as presents. If they give the muscletoe as a gift, they must also give the person information about the muscle.

★ *MUSCLETOE SECRET:* If you see someone standing underneath the muscletoe, give him or her a hug.

SAFETY CONSIDERATIONS

Be careful to prevent falls from a ladder or chair when hanging up the muscletoe around the school.

ADAPTATION SUGGESTIONS

If you don't want the whole class to make muscletoe, use the activity as a reward. Students who have earned a reward can make one to decorate the school, give to a friend or parents, or keep for themselves.

TEACHING HINTS

Younger children will probably need help making their muscletoe.

Give students information about mistletoe so they can see the humor in making muscletoe.

Hanukkah Dreidel Game

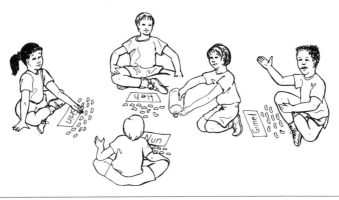

Figure 4.7 Hanukkah dreidel game.

QUICK DESCRIPTION

A quiet, small-group game (Figure 4.7)

APPROPRIATE GRADES

K-6

ACTIVITY GOALS

To learn the story of Hanukkah and how to play the dreidel game

SPACE REQUIRED

Gymnasium, classroom, or outside area

KEY SKILLS

Working cooperatively in a small group and following game rules

EQUIPMENT AND PREPARATION

Collect **1 empty 2-liter soda bottle for every 5 students** in your class. Make **a set of game cards** for each group of four students. You can make the game cards out of index cards. Each set of four cards should include the following:

- Nun (N)—The player gets nothing.
- Gimel (G)—The player takes all.
- Heh (H)—The player takes half.
- Shin (Sh)—The player puts one in.

You will also need **10 or more small game pieces for each student**, such as beans, pennies, or pea gravel.

ACTIVITY PROCEDURE

Before the students play the game, discuss Hanukkah with them. Your school library probably has a book about Hanukkah. An old custom connected with Hanukkah is a game called the *Dreidel*. A dreidel is a four-sided top. A Hebrew letter is engraved on each of the four sides. The letters are Nun (N), Gimel (G), Heh (H), and Shin (Sh). These letters stand for the Hebrew words *nes gadol hayah sham*, which means *a great miracle took place there*. They also stand for the Yiddish-German words *nem* (take), *gib* (give), *halb* (half), and *shtel tzu* (add).

Divide the class into groups of five. Distribute any extra students among the groups. Students should sit on the floor when then play the game. Each group makes a circle of students with one student in the center. Give each of the students in the circle one of the game cards to place on the floor in front of them. Give the students in the center a 2-liter soda bottle. The student in the center is the spinner. Give each student 10 game pieces.

The game is played as follows:

Each player puts one game piece in the center. Then the center student spins the bottle. When it stops, the student it is pointing to reads the game card and the student in the center follows those directions. He or she will either take none of the game pieces in the center, take all the pieces in the center, take half the pieces, or put one game piece in. This procedure is repeated with a different student as the spinner. The previous spinner exchanges places with the new spinner. The student with the most game pieces when the time is up is the winner.

SAFETY CONSIDERATIONS

Tell students not to throw the game pieces or the bottles.

ADAPTATION SUGGESTIONS

If you would like to add some movement to the game, the spinner can lead an exercise before spinning the bottle.

TEACHING HINTS

Please teach your students about Hanukkah and the dreidel so they can understand and respect the Jewish tradition. Ask the students if any of them are familiar with the story of Hanukkah or the Dreidel game. If they are, have them tell the story or explain the game.

This is a good game to play as a cool-down during the holidays.

Blizzard

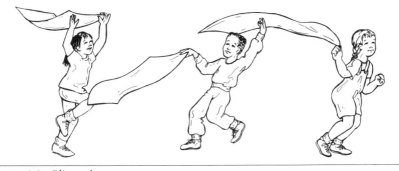

Figure 4.8 Blizzard.

QUICK DESCRIPTION

A manipulative, creative, rhythmic activity or aerobic dance (Figure 4.8)

APPROPRIATE GRADES

K-6

ACTIVITY GOALS

To perform the manipulative skills correctly with plastic sheets to the beat of the music, and to create a dance using the skills

SPACE REQUIRED

Gymnasium

KEY SKILLS

Various locomotor and nonlocomotor skills

EQUIPMENT AND PREPARATION

You will need **a piece of white material for each student**. Cut-open white plastic trash bags work great. Choose some **"blizzard" music**. The "Tornado" from *The Wiz* is a favorite. Classical music is also a good choice. You will also need **a record or cassette player**.

ACTIVITY PROCEDURE

Have students perform the following activities with the plastic sheets, first without and then with music:

• Hold one corner of the plastic sheet in each hand above the head and walk, run, gallop, skip, leap, jump, hop, and slide

• Hold the sheet in one hand and walk, run, gallop, skip, leap, jump, hop, and slide; students should practice with both their right and left hands

• Hold one corner of the sheet in each hand and wave it up and down; have students try to do this slowly and quickly

• Hold the sheet in one hand and wave it up and down; have students try to do this slowly and quickly—they should also practice with both their right and left hands

• Make designs in space using both hands to hold the sheet, then the right hand only, then the left hand only; make the designs in front of the body, over the head, and out to the sides—have students try to make shapes, numbers, and letters

• Swing, shake, and twist the sheet

• Throw the sheet up into the air either crumbled up like a ball or opened up, and perform different movements before the sheet comes down, such as clapping, turning around, jumping, hopping, sitting down, and lying down; after practicing these movements to the music, play the music again and let the students create their own "blizzard" dances

SAFETY CONSIDERATIONS

Tell the students not to put the plastic sheet over their faces, in their mouths, or around their necks. Stress that students watch out for each other to avoid collisions.

ADAPTATION SUGGESTIONS

Older children may not be as willing to do creative dance as younger ones. Instead, you can make an aerobic dance routine out of this activity.

TEACHING HINTS

When the children are creating their own dances, watch for children who run very fast no matter the speed of the music and for children who like to chase others. If they continue to do these things, have them sit out for a while and watch the children that are following the directions correctly.

Skateless Skating

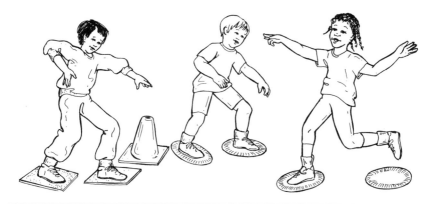

Figure 4.9 Skateless skating.

QUICK DESCRIPTION

Manipulative rhythmic locomotor activity using carpet squares or paper plates (Figure 4.9)

APPROPRIATE GRADES

K-6

ACTIVITY GOALS

To move (skate) with a carpet square or paper plate under each foot in a variety of situations, such as to music, through obstacles, or in a game

SPACE REQUIRED

Gymnasium

KEY SKILLS

Manipulating carpet squares with feet to move forward, backward, sideways, and to turn around; and performing these skills to music, through obstacles, and in a game situation

EQUIPMENT AND PREPARATION

You will need **2 paper plates or carpet squares** for each student, **16 traffic cones** or other obstacles, **a record or cassette** ("Skaters' Waltz" is great), and **a record or cassette player**.

ACTIVITY PROCEDURE

Demonstrate how students should move to avoid losing their skates. Have the students perform the following activities using two carpet squares or paper plates as skates:

- Skate forward, backward, right, and left, and turn to the right and left

- Skate forward, backward, right, left, and turn to the right and left, while listening to music

- Create a skating routine to music

- Arrange the students in four rows and arrange four rows of cones for them to skate through

- Older children can have skating relay races

- Simple games such as tag can be played while wearing the skates

SAFETY CONSIDERATIONS

Emphasize that students try to stay on their feet and not fall down purposely when skating. Stress that they avoid collisions by watching out for other children when they are skating.

ADAPTATION SUGGESTIONS

Older children will prefer to participate in relay races and games while wearing the skates.

TEACHING HINTS

Explain that students must slide their feet along the floor to keep their skates on. If they lift up their feet they will lose their skates.

Chapter 5

FEBRUARY

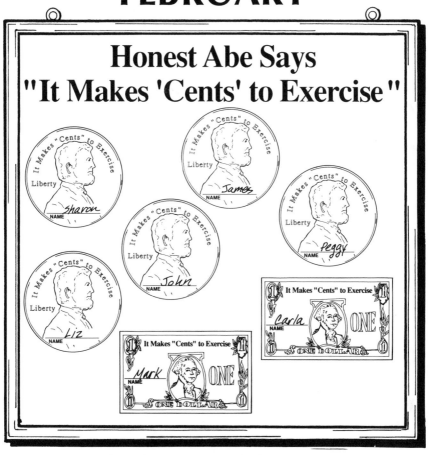

Honest Abe Says
"It Makes 'Cents' to Exercise"

VALENTINE'S DAY,
PRESIDENTS' DAY,
GROUNDHOG DAY

Honest Abe—
It Makes "Cents" to Exercise

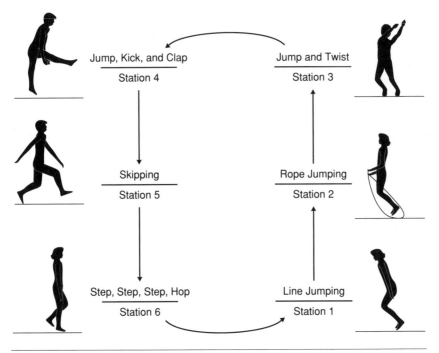

Figure 5.1 Honest Abe—It makes "cents" to exercise.

QUICK DESCRIPTION
Aerobic exercise circuit training course (Figure 5.1)

APPROPRIATE GRADES
K-6

ACTIVITY GOALS
To improve physical fitness levels, especially cardiovascular endurance, by motivating students to put more effort into the physical fitness exercises

SPACE REQUIRED
Gymnasium, track, or large outside area

KEY SKILLS
The February circuit training course includes the following skills to help improve cardiovascular endurance:

- *Line Jumping*—Students continuously jump from side to side or forward and backward over a line taped on the floor.

- *Rope Jumping*—Students jump rope continuously.

- *Jump and Twist*—Students jump in place continuously while twisting the body from side to side.

- *Jump, Kick, and Clap*—Students kick the right leg forward while clapping hands underneath, and then repeat with left leg. Students should keep alternating between their right and left legs.

- *Skipping*—Students skip continuously in a small area.

- *Step, Step, Step, Hop*—Students step R-L-R and hop R, and then step L-R-L and hop L. Repeat continuously.

Students also walk briskly.

EQUIPMENT AND PREPARATION

Start this circuit training course at the beginning of February. For the sample circuit training course, construct **7 signs**, one for each of the exercise stations and one that says "Honest Abe Says It Makes 'Cents' to Exercise." The station signs should be "Line Jumping," "Rope Jumping," "Jump and Twist," "Jump, Kick, and Clap," "Skipping," and "Step, Step, Step, Hop." Reproduce enough **"It Makes 'Cents' to Exercise" certificates** (Figure A.11a in the appendix) for everyone in your class.

You will need **a record or cassette player** and **a record or cassette** of a lively piece of music that the students will like. Some suggestions are "At the Hop" (Danny and the Juniors, MCA Records), "Rock Around the Clock" (Bill Haley and the Comets, Decca Records), or "Tequila" (The Champs, Masters International Inc.). You will also need **6 traffic cones**, one to designate the location of each station.

Attach the "Honest Abe Says It Makes 'Cents' to Exercise" sign to the wall or bulletin board where everyone can see and set up the exercise stations.

Build excitement and interest by putting up signs around the school about a week before that say "You Can Earn 'Cents' by Exercising" or "I'd Bet That Honest Abe Did All of His Exercises!"

ACTIVITY PROCEDURE

Review the activity procedures for circuit training courses on page xii. Give the signal to start, and play the music. Allow about 15 seconds for each station.

Students earn an "Honest Abe Says It Makes 'Cents' to Exercise" certificate the first time they correctly complete the course and a small cherry drawn on their certificate each time they complete the course after that. When students have completed the course a designated number of times, they earn a dollar bill certificate with George Washington's picture on it (Figure A.11b in the appendix).

SAFETY CONSIDERATIONS

Tell students to exercise at a level where they feel comfortable. They don't have to overdo it.

ADAPTATION SUGGESTIONS

Many other aerobic activities can be used at the stations to fit your students' needs.

TEACHING HINTS

Tell students that it is more important that they perform the circuit without stopping, even if they must go a little slower, than to perform the exercises very hard and fast and later end up stopping. Duration is more important than intensity.

Groundhog Maze and Shadow Play

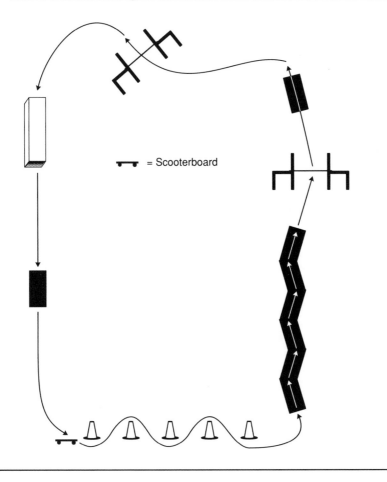

= Scooterboard

Shadow play area

Figure 5.2 Groundhog maze and shadow play.

QUICK DESCRIPTION
Obstacle course and shadow-movement activity (Figure 5.2)

APPROPRIATE GRADES
K-6

ACTIVITY GOALS
To complete the skills in the obstacle course correctly by trusting and cooperating with a partner, and to develop creativity while making their own shadows move on the wall

SPACE REQUIRED

Gymnasium

KEY SKILLS

Developing trust and cooperation between partners in order to complete the skills in the course while blindfolded

EQUIPMENT AND PREPARATION

Reproduce enough **"I Saw My Shadow" certificates** (Figure A.12 in the appendix) for everyone in your class. Make arrangements to use the **overhead projector**. Get two if possible. Assemble the obstacle course. You will also need some or all of the following equipment: **blindfolds for half of the class**, enough **tumbling mats to make 2 tunnels, 2 more mats, obstacles to go under and over** (a stick between two chairs works well), and **5 traffic cones**.

Motivate the students by putting up signs around the school about a week before the activity that say "Will You See Your Shadow in Physical Education Class?" or "Will You Escape the Groundhog's Maze?"

ACTIVITY PROCEDURE

Review the activity procedures for obstacle courses on page xiii. Explain the obstacle course. About half the students are groundhogs and are blindfolded. The groundhogs' partners must lead them through the course safely to the shadow play area. The groundhogs are not allowed to peek. They are supposed to follow the directions given to them by their partners. When they have reached the shadow play area safely, they may remove the blindfolds and experiment by making shadows for a few minutes. Then the partners change places. Students who trust their partners and complete the course without peeking receive an "I Saw My Shadow" certificate.

These are the activities included in the sample course:

- walking through a maze made from mats
- going under an obstacle (a stick between two chairs)
- performing a crab walk across a mat
- going over an obstacle (a low stick between two chairs)
- crawling through a tunnel made from mats
- performing a log roll across a mat
- maneuvering through traffic cones while sitting on a scooterboard

SAFETY CONSIDERATIONS

Keep the activities simple, because the students will be performing them blindfolded. Stress that the leader is responsible for the other student's safety while traveling through the obstacle course. The blindfolded students should feel that they can trust their partners to lead them through the course safely. The leaders should guide their partners mainly by talking. Younger children can also guide by touching if they don't know right from left.

ADAPTATION SUGGESTIONS

Let the younger students participate in the obstacle course a few times without being blindfolded so they can become familiar with it. You may want to eliminate the scooterboard activity for younger children.

TEACHING HINTS

The leaders should tell the blindfolded students which activity is next before the students get to it.

Healthy Heart
and Valentine's Day Skills Stations

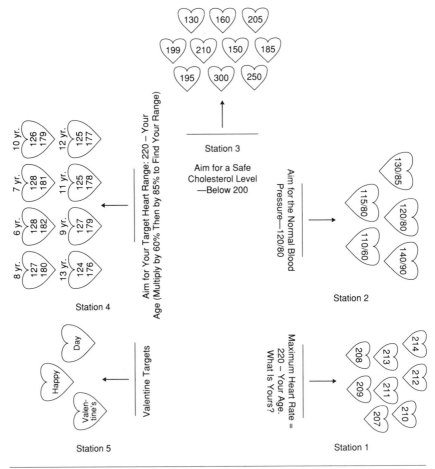

Figure 5.3 Healthy heart and Valentine's Day stations.

QUICK DESCRIPTION

Throwing skills stations and heart information (Figure 5.3)

APPROPRIATE GRADES

3-6

ACTIVITY GOALS

To improve throwing for accuracy while learning about the heart

SPACE REQUIRED

Gymnasium

KEY SKILLS

Overhand throwing and demonstrating knowledge of maximum heart rate, target heart rate, safe cholesterol level, and normal blood pressure

EQUIPMENT AND PREPARATION

For the five stations you will need to do the following:

• *Maximum Heart Rate*—Make **a sign** that says "Maximum Heart Rate = 220 – Your Age. What Is Yours?" and **small paper hearts** with different heart-rate numbers on each.

• *Blood Pressure*—Make **a sign** that says "Aim for the Normal Blood Pressure—120/80" and **small paper hearts** with different blood-pressure readings on each.

• *Cholesterol*—Make **a sign** that says "Aim for a Safe Cholesterol Level—Below 200" and **small paper hearts** with different cholesterol levels on each.

• *Target Heart Rate*—Make **a sign** that says "Aim for Your Target Heart Range: 220 – Your Age (Multiply by 60% and Then by 85% to Find Your Range)" and **small paper hearts** with different heart rates on each.

• *Valentine Targets*—Make **3 paper hearts** that say "Happy," "Valentine's," and "Day." Set up the stations.

You will also need **5 beanbags** and enough **paper and pencils** for everyone in the class.

ACTIVITY PROCEDURE

Review the activity procedures for skills stations on page xiv. Explain each station to the class.

Station Description

• *Maximum Heart Rate*—Students calculate their maximum heart rate and throw beanbags at the paper heart with their number on it. Have paper and pencils available for the students.

• *Blood Pressure*—Students aim for the paper heart that has the numbers for normal blood pressure on it (120/80).

• *Cholesterol*—Students aim for the paper heart that has the number below which their cholesterol level should be (200).

- *Target Heart Rate*—Students calculate their target heart rate's low and high range (60% and 85%), and aim for the paper hearts with those numbers.
- *Valentine Targets*—Students aim for the words "Happy Valentine's Day" in the correct order.

SAFETY CONSIDERATIONS

Leave ample space between the stations. Tell students not to stand in the throwing area.

ADAPTATION SUGGESTIONS

If third graders are not able to do some of the calculations, tell them what their maximum and target heart rates should be. Children in grades lower than third can practice throwing skills using the Valentine targets.

TEACHING HINTS

Review maximum heart rate, target heart rate, cholesterol level, and blood pressure before the students participate in the stations.

Throwing Across the Potomac

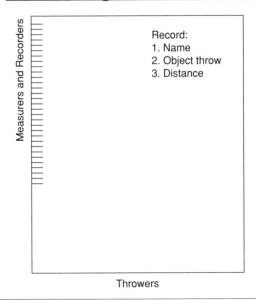

Figure 5.4   Throwing across the Potomac.

QUICK DESCRIPTION

Throwing for distance (Figure 5.4)

APPROPRIATE GRADES

K-6

ACTIVITY GOALS

To increase the distance an object can be thrown and to be able to measure that distance and to work cooperatively in a small group

SPACE REQUIRED

Large outside area or gymnasium

KEY SKILLS

Overhand throwing for distance, and measuring

EQUIPMENT AND PREPARATION

Mark off the outside area or gymnasium in 1-foot increments. You can do this with **traffic cones**. Place the first cone at the 10-foot mark and continue from there. You will need various types of **balls, flying disks, or other objects for throwing; a tape measure; tape or a long rope** to mark the throwing line; and **1 pencil and 1 piece of paper for every 3 students.**

ACTIVITY PROCEDURE

Review the correct way to perform the overhand throw. Divide the class as evenly as possible into groups of three and give each student in each group a number—1, 2, or 3. Student 1 will be George Washington (the thrower), Student 2 will be the measurer, and Student 3 will record the score. Each group chooses the object they want to throw. The thrower in each group stands behind the throwing line. The throwers should spread out as much as possible. If your class is very large, you may have to limit the number of students throwing at once. The measurer stands out in the field but may not interfere with the objects that are being thrown. The recorder stands off to the side. The thrower takes three consecutive turns, the measurer tells the thrower and the recorder the distances thrown, and the recorder writes the scores down on the paper. The distance is measured from the throwing line to the spot where the object first touches the ground, not to where it rolls or bounces. Then Student 2 becomes the thrower, Student 3 becomes the measurer, and Student 1 becomes the recorder. This procedure repeats until all three students have performed each job. Then the group chooses a different object to throw and the entire throwing, measuring, and recording sequence repeats. Make sure the recorders write down the thrower's name, the object being thrown, and the distances.

SAFETY CONSIDERATIONS

If you do this activity in the gymnasium, restrict the types of objects to be thrown. Flying disks and hard balls should be saved for outside. Stress that students do not interfere with the objects being thrown.

ADAPTATION SUGGESTIONS

If you don't have a large area, use objects that don't travel as far, such as sponge balls. You can specify a certain distance the ball must travel across the Potomac River. Younger students may need for the first cone to be closer than 10 feet, and they may not be able to measure and record on their own.

TEACHING HINTS

Emphasize that using correct throwing form makes the objects travel farther.

Broken Hearts

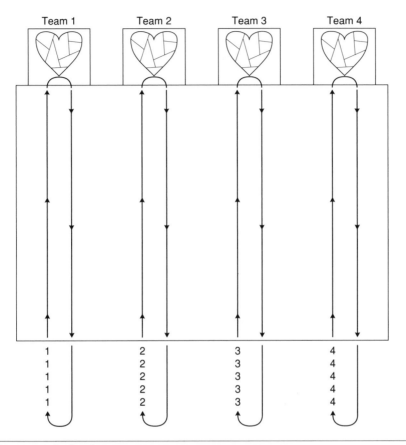

Figure 5.5 Broken hearts.

QUICK DESCRIPTION
Cooperative relay race (Figure 5.5)

APPROPRIATE GRADES
K-6

ACTIVITY GOALS
To perform the locomotor skills correctly, to work cooperatively in a group, and to demonstrate knowledge of game and safety rules in a game situation

SPACE REQUIRED
Gymnasium

KEY SKILLS

Various locomotor skills such as running, galloping, skipping, and animal walking; participating cooperatively in a group; obeying the rules of a game; and demonstrating knowledge of safety rules while playing a game

EQUIPMENT AND PREPARATION

You will need **4 or 5 different Valentine pictures** (you can purchase these at any card shop around Valentine's Day). The number of pictures depends on the number of relay teams you will have. Laminate the pictures to protect them, and then cut them into equal pieces so there is at least one piece for every student on each team. If you buy the type that has a picture on both sides, mark each piece on one of the sides so that the students won't have reversed pieces. You will also need **1 small container for each puzzle** (turned-over flying disks work fine).

ACTIVITY PROCEDURE

Explain the relay race to the class. Divide the class, as evenly as possible, into relay teams. Arrange the teams in single-file lines at one end of the gym behind a starting line. You can make a line with masking tape if there is no line painted on the gym floor. At the other end of the gym, place a container with the puzzle pieces even with each team. On the signal, the first student in each line performs the designated locomotor skill while approaching the container, takes one puzzle piece from the container, returns to the starting line, and tags right hands with the next team member. This procedure continues until all of the puzzle pieces have been retrieved from the container. As the race is in progress, team members work together to put the puzzle pieces together. The first team that finishes the puzzle correctly is the winner. Teams can exchange puzzles and race again.

SAFETY CONSIDERATIONS

Place the starting line and containers a safe distance from walls to avoid accidents. Also, stress that students tag right hands to avoid collisions. Don't allow the students to slide to the finish line.

ADAPTATION SUGGESTIONS

You can make the puzzles easier by purchasing two of each of the Valentine pictures. Cut up one for the puzzle, and give the other to each team as a model for putting the pieces together. For a more difficult puzzle, you can cut red hearts from construction paper and laminate them. Then cut each heart into equal pieces and mark one of the sides. Vary the locomotor skills used according to ability.

TEACHING HINTS

Make sure each team knows which container is theirs to avoid confusion when the race starts. It's a good idea to walk each team through the race procedure first.

This is a good relay because even a team that is lagging behind in the race can win if they put the puzzle together quickly. Stress cooperation.

Heart Potato

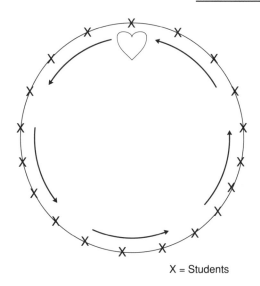

X = Students

Figure 5.6   Heart potato.

QUICK DESCRIPTION

Musical aerobic exercise game (Figure 5.6)

APPROPRIATE GRADES

K-6

ACTIVITY GOALS

To lead the class in an aerobic movement and to follow game rules

SPACE REQUIRED

Gymnasium

KEY SKILLS

Moving aerobically to the rhythm of the music, leading a group, and following game rules

EQUIPMENT AND PREPARATION

You will need **a record or cassette player** and some **lively music** that the students will enjoy (marches are great for the younger children). Cut **a large heart out of red construction paper** and laminate it. You could also purchase a very large, inflatable Valentine heart. The students will love it!

ACTIVITY PROCEDURE

Arrange the class in a circle. Explain the game to the students. Play the music and demonstrate a few movements that the students could do if they are caught with the "Heart Potato." Tell them that you would rather have them create their own movements than repeat the ones you did. Give the heart to one of the students. When the music begins, this student passes the heart to the student next to him or her. The passing continues until the music stops. The student who is holding the heart when the music stops goes to the center of the circle and performs an aerobic movement to the music. Play the music again. The whole class performs the movement until you say stop. Then the students continue passing the heart around the circle where they left off. This procedure continues until you stop the activity.

SAFETY CONSIDERATIONS

When you make the circle, leave some space between the students so they don't accidentally hit each other when they are exercising. Tell them to hand the heart to the student next to them and not to throw it. Also tell the students that they must stay on their feet.

ADAPTATION SUGGESTIONS

You can use different types of music with various age groups.

TEACHING HINTS

Make leading the exercises a reward, not a punishment. Say things like "Who will be the lucky one to lead the exercise when the music stops?" Do not say "If you get stuck with the heart you have to lead an exercise."

There probably won't be enough time for all the students to lead an exercise in one class period. You can use the game as their exercise during a few class sessions so they can all have a chance to lead. Have the students walk around the gym for a few minutes to cool down.

Chapter 6

MARCH

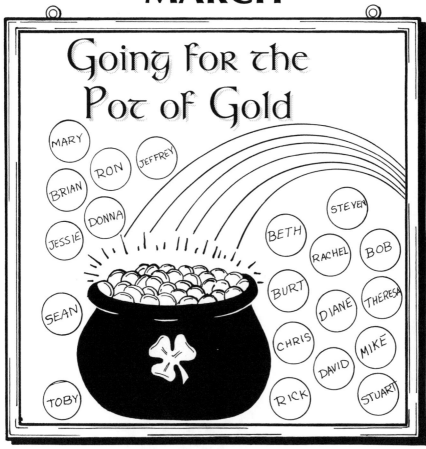

Going for the
Pot of Gold

MARY
RON
JEFFREY
BRIAN
DONNA
JESSIE
SEAN
TOBY
STEVEN
BETH
RACHEL
BOB
BURT
DIANE
THERESA
CHRIS
DAVID
MIKE
RICK
STUART

ST. PATRICK'S DAY

Going for the Pot of Gold

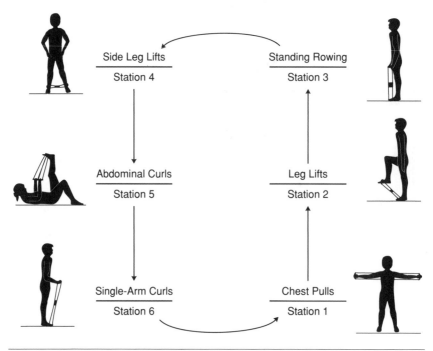

Figure 6.1 Going for the pot of gold.

QUICK DESCRIPTION

Physical fitness exercise circuit training course (Figure 6.1)

APPROPRIATE GRADES

K-6

ACTIVITY GOALS

To improve physical fitness levels, especially muscular strength and endurance and cardiovascular endurance, by motivating the students to put more effort into the physical fitness exercises

SPACE REQUIRED

Gymnasium, track, or large outside area

KEY SKILLS

The March circuit training course emphasizes the following skills:

- Chest and arm strength and endurance (chest pulls)
- Leg strength and endurance (leg lifts, side leg lifts)

- Shoulder girdle strength and endurance (standing rowing)
- Abdominal strength and endurance (abdominal curls)
- Arm strength and endurance (single-arm curls)
- Cardiovascular endurance (skipping)

EQUIPMENT AND PREPARATION

Start this circuit training course at the beginning of March. For the sample circuit training course, construct **7 signs**, one for each of the exercise stations and one that says "Going for the Pot of Gold." The station signs should be "Chest Pulls," "Leg Lifts," "Standing Rowing," "Side Leg Lifts," "Abdominal Curls," and "Single-Arm Curls." Using gold construction paper, cut enough **circles** (gold pieces) for everyone in your class. Also cut **a pot** for the gold out of black construction paper. Add **a rainbow** in the background to make it complete. You could use different colored chalk on a large piece of paper.

Attach the "Going for the Pot of Gold" sign, the pot, and the rainbow to a wall or bulletin board, and set up the exercise stations. You will need **1 exercise rubber band or piece of medical latex tubing for each student in the class.**

You will also need **a record or cassette player** and **a lively Irish song**, such as "McNamara's Band," for exercise music.

Build excitement and interest by putting up signs around the school that say "Will You Get the Gold in Physical Education Class?" or "Will You Be a Lucky Leprechaun in Physical Education Class?"

ACTIVITY PROCEDURE

Review the activity procedures for circuit training courses on page xii. Allow about 15 seconds for each station. Students earn a personalized paper gold piece the first time they complete the course. Draw a shamrock on it each time they complete the course after that.

SAFETY CONSIDERATIONS

Tell the students to hold the rubber bands tightly so they don't accidentally snap themselves or other students with them. They should also make sure that the rubberbands are kept away from the skipping area to avoid accidents.

ADAPTATION SUGGESTIONS

If you do not have enough exercise rubber bands for each student, choose different exercises for the stations.

TEACHING HINTS

Make sure the students have had previous instruction in the use of the exercise rubber bands. Choose exercises with which they are familiar.

I'm Climbing
Over a Four-Leaf Clover

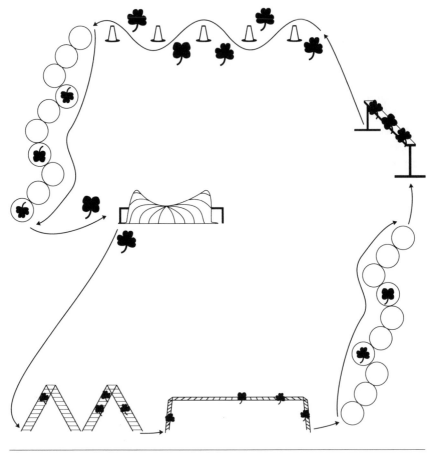

Figure 6.2   I'm climbing over a four-leaf clover.

QUICK DESCRIPTION
Obstacle course (Figure 6.2)

APPROPRIATE GRADES
K-6

ACTIVITY GOALS
To complete the skills in the obstacle course correctly while counting four-leaf clovers along the way

SPACE REQUIRED

Gymnasium

KEY SKILLS

Showing bodily control while performing the obstacle course; demonstrating perceptual motor skills; jumping into hoops; hopping into hoops; dribbling a basketball through cones; climbing over ladders or other obstacles; maneuvering under obstacles; hanging and traveling on a horizontal ladder; and walking backwards on the balance beam

EQUIPMENT AND PREPARATION

Reproduce **20 or more shamrocks** (Figure A.13a in the appendix) and about **10 four-leaf clovers** (Figure A.13b in the appendix). Also reproduce enough **"Luck of the Irish" certificates** (Figure A.13c in the appendix) for everyone in your class. Assemble the obstacle course and attach shamrocks and four-leaf clovers in various places. You will need some or all of the following: **12 or more Hula Hoops, a few basketballs, 5 traffic cones, obstacles to travel under** (a parachute draped over a chair works fine), **ladders or other obstacles for climbing, a horizontal ladder, a balance beam**, and enough **mats** to put around the equipment.

Motivate the students by putting up signs around the school about a week before the event is held that say "How Many Lucky Four-Leaf Clovers Will You Find in Physical Education Class?" or "The Leprechauns Have Been Busy Hiding Shamrocks and Four-Leaf Clovers in the Gym. Will You Find Them All?"

ACTIVITY PROCEDURE

Review the activity procedures for obstacle courses on page xiii. Explain the obstacle course to the class. The performers silently count four-leaf clovers along the way so that the partners don't hear the number of four-leaf clovers. When everyone has had a turn, ask the students how many four-leaf clovers they counted. Students with the correct number whose partners say that they performed the skills correctly, receive a "Luck of the Irish" certificate.

These activities are included in the sample course:

• Hula Hoops are placed on the floor. Students jump from one hoop to another without stepping on them.

• Students walk backwards on the balance beam.

• Students dribble a basketball through traffic cones.

• Hula Hoops are placed on the floor. Students hop on one foot from one hoop to another without stepping on them.

- Students move under a parachute draped over some chairs without touching it.

- Students climb over ladders or other obstacles.

- Students hang from rungs on a horizontal ladder and travel from one end to the other.

SAFETY CONSIDERATIONS

Emphasize that students begin on the signal and stop when they complete the course. Place an adequate number of mats around the balance beam, horizontal ladder, climbing ladders, and any other area where they are necessary.

ADAPTATION SUGGESTIONS

Vary the activities according to the skill level of the children. The activities can be adapted for children with disabilities.

TEACHING HINTS

Choose activities with which the children are familiar.

Lucky Leprechaun Skills Stations

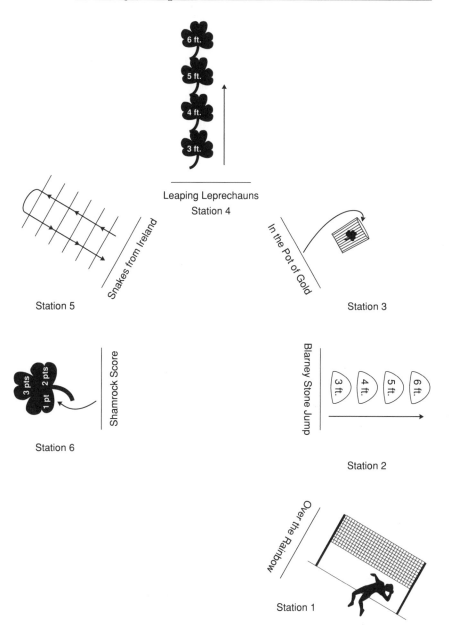

Figure 6.3 Lucky leprechaun stations.

QUICK DESCRIPTION

Locomotor skills stations and throwing practice (Figure 6.3)

APPROPRIATE GRADES

K-6

ACTIVITY GOALS

To improve skill level in throwing, jumping, leaping, and hopping

SPACE REQUIRED

Gymnasium

KEY SKILLS

Underhand throwing, overhand throwing, throwing the flying disk, performing the standing long jump, leaping, and hopping

EQUIPMENT AND PREPARATION

For the six stations you will need to do the following:

• *Over the Rainbow*—Make **a sign** that says "Over The Rainbow" and set up **a volleyball net or a rope** for the students to throw over. Provide **2 yellow or gold flying disks.**

• *Blarney Stone Jump*—Make **a sign** that says "Blarney Stone Jump" and about **6 Blarney stones** (ovals cut from brown construction paper with distances on them). Tape the stones to the floor. You will also need **a tape measure.**

• *In the Pot of Gold*—Make **a sign** that says "In the Pot of Gold." You will need **2 yellow or gold beanbags** and **1 trash barrel or box.**

• *Leaping Leprechauns*—Make **a sign** that says "Leaping Leprechauns" and **6 small shamrocks** with distances marked on them (Figure A.13a in the appendix). Tape the shamrocks to the floor. You will also need **a tape measure.**

• *Snakes from Ireland*—Make **a sign** that says "Snakes From Ireland." You will also need **6 jump ropes.**

• *Shamrock Score*—Make **a sign** that says "Shamrock Score" and **a large shamrock** to use as a target. Write the numbers 1, 2, and 3 on the three sections of the shamrock. You will also need **2 beanbags.**

Set up the stations.

ACTIVITY PROCEDURE

Review the activity procedures for skills stations on page xiv. Explain each station to the class.

Station Description

- *Over the Rainbow*—Students throw "gold" flying disks over a volleyball net. They score a point if the disk doesn't touch the net when it goes over.
- *Blarney Stone Jump*—Students perform a standing long jump. The Blarney stones mark the distances they have jumped.
- *In the Pot of Gold*—Students throw gold-colored beanbags or balls into a trash barrel or box. Students earn a point for each successful throw.
- *Leaping Leprechauns*—Students leap as far as they can. The shamrocks mark the distances.
- *Snakes From Ireland*—Arrange jump ropes in rows on the floor. Students must hop over them and back without stepping on them or putting down their non-hopping foot.
- *Shamrock Score*—Students throw overhand at the shamrock target. They can earn 1, 2, or 3 points, depending on the number they hit.

SAFETY CONSIDERATIONS

Tell students not to crowd the person who is taking a turn. You may want to use a mat for the standing long jump if students are falling backwards after they jump.

ADAPTATION SUGGESTIONS

Shorten or lengthen the distance from the throwing line to the target depending on skill level.

Students can keep score on paper if desired.

TEACHING HINTS

Teach the skills to the students before they practice at the stations.

Windy March

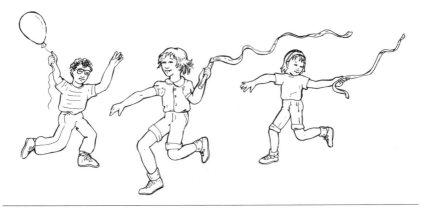

Figure 6.4 Windy March.

QUICK DESCRIPTION
Outside activities with ribbons, streamers, and balloons (Figure 6.4)

APPROPRIATE GRADES
K-3

ACTIVITY GOALS
To improve cardiovascular endurance by motivating students to exercise longer

SPACE REQUIRED
Large outside area or track

KEY SKILLS
Running, jogging, and pacing

EQUIPMENT AND PREPARATION
You will need **a ribbon attached to a stick, a streamer, or a balloon on a string for each student**. If you use balloons, inflate them and tie on the string.

If you do only relays and not the continuous aerobic exercise, you will only need a ribbon, streamer, or a balloon on a string and a traffic cone for each team, not for each student.

Note: "Super balloons" are 10-foot-long plastic balloons. When you hold the end open and run with them, they inflate until you stop running. They cost about a dollar each and motivate the children to run continuously for a very long time. You may be able to find them at a carnival supply store. The children really enjoy them.

ACTIVITY PROCEDURE

Aerobic Activity

The whole class can do this activity at the same time. Explain that the students will jog continuously for as long as they can. If they get tired they may walk for a while and then start jogging again. Tell them to hold their ribbon, streamer, or balloon up in the air so it flies in the wind.

Relay Race

Explain the relay race to the class. Divide the class, as evenly as possible, into four relay teams. Arrange the teams in single-file lines at one end of the field behind a starting line. Give the first person in each row a ribbon, streamer, or balloon on a string. At the other end of the field, place a traffic cone for each team to designate the turning point.

On the signal, the first person on each team runs with the ribbon, streamer, or balloon down to the traffic cone. He or she goes around the cone and returns to the starting line. The runner hands the ribbon, streamer, or balloon to the next student (who takes his or her turn exactly as the first student did), and goes to the end of the line. This procedure continues until everyone on each team has had a turn. The first team to finish, wins. If the teams are uneven, have someone run twice. Choose a different student to run twice each time.

SAFETY CONSIDERATIONS

In the relay, place the starting line and cones a safe distance from walls and fences to avoid accidents. Students should pass the ribbons, streamers, and balloons with right hands to avoid collisions.

ADAPTATION SUGGESTIONS

You can take your class on an exercise walk, possibly through the neighborhood, with their ribbons, streamers, or balloons.

You can use a variety of locomotor skills for the relays.

TEACHING HINTS

Ask some older students to inflate the balloons and tie strings on them for you.

For the aerobic activity, stress that the students pace themselves when jogging. Many students, especially the younger ones, run very fast, tire quickly, and end up walking.

For relays, make sure each team knows which traffic cone is theirs. It's a good idea to walk each team through the relay procedure first so there is no confusion.

Lions and Lambs

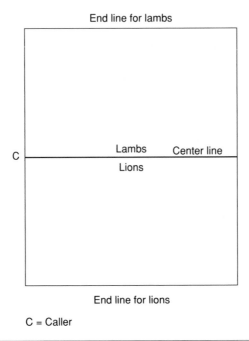

End line for lambs

C

Lambs   Center line

Lions

End line for lions

C = Caller

Figure 6.5 Lions and lambs.

QUICK DESCRIPTION

A chasing and fleeing game (Figure 6.5)

APPROPRIATE GRADES

K-3

ACTIVITY GOALS

To demonstrate bodily control and knowledge of game and safety rules in a game situation

SPACE REQUIRED

Large outside area or gymnasium

KEY SKILLS

Running, chasing, fleeing, dodging, and tagging safely; and developing honesty and good sportsmanship

EQUIPMENT AND PREPARATION

Mark off a large playing area with two end lines and a center line. Use traffic cones if necessary.

ACTIVITY PROCEDURE

Divide the class, as evenly as possible, into two groups—the lions and the lambs. Tell the students to line up back to back on the center dividing line. Then have them take three steps away from each other. Choose one student to be the caller. When the game begins, the caller, who tries to fool both teams about whom he or she will call, shouts either "l-l-l-lions" or "l-l-l-lambs." If the caller says "lions," the lions chase the lambs to their goal line, trying to catch as many as they can. If the caller says "lambs," then the lambs chase the lions to their goal line. Students count the number of lions or lambs they catch. Then both groups return to their original starting positions, a new caller is chosen, and the game begins again.

SAFETY CONSIDERATIONS

Emphasize that the students tag lightly when they try to catch someone. They should not push each other or grab clothing.

Keep the goal line a safe distance from walls or fences so the students don't run into them. When outside, play on grass rather than blacktop to avoid cuts and scrapes if students fall.

Make sure there are at least 6 feet between the two groups at the beginning of each game to prevent collisions when the group turns around to chase.

ADAPTATION SUGGESTIONS

Adapt the size of the playing area to each class.

The game can also be played with the two groups facing each other instead of standing back to back.

TEACHING HINTS

Stress that students play fairly and be honest when they are tagged.

Blarney Stone Tag

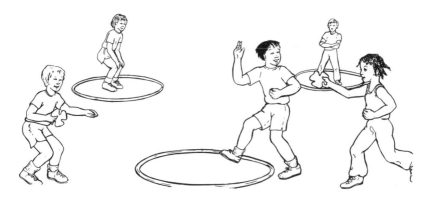

Figure 6.6 Blarney stone tag.

QUICK DESCRIPTION
A chasing and fleeing game (Figure 6.6)

APPROPRIATE GRADES
K-6

ACTIVITY GOALS
To demonstrate bodily control and knowledge of game and safety rules in a game situation

SPACE REQUIRED
Gymnasium or outside area with marked boundaries

KEY SKILLS
Running, dodging, and tagging safely; and developing honesty and good sportsmanship

EQUIPMENT AND PREPARATION
Reproduce **a few paper shamrocks** (Figure A.13a in the appendix). Tape **6 bases or Hula Hoops** to the floor in a scattered pattern.

ACTIVITY PROCEDURE
Choose one to four students to be "it." These students are the leprechauns and each one carries a paper shamrock with which to tag. Well-defined boundaries are needed for the game whether it is played inside or outside. If a player goes outside the boundaries, he or she is considered tagged. During the game, the Blarney stones (bases or hoops) are safety zones.

Only one player may stand on a Blarney stone at a time. When a player is tagged, the leprechaun hands over the shamrock and the tagged player becomes "it."

SAFETY CONSIDERATIONS

Emphasize that the students tag lightly with the shamrock. They should tag on arms, legs, back, or chest, and not the face. Students must not push or grab clothing when trying to tag someone.

Keep boundaries away from walls or fences to avoid accidents. Clear the playing area of dangerous objects, such as chairs, tables, and other equipment. Tape the hoops to the floor so the students don't slip while playing.

ADAPTATION SUGGESTIONS

Provide extra Blarney stones when younger children are playing so they can rest more.

Older children can keep score by counting the number of times they are tagged. Those students tagged the least amount of times, win.

TEACHING HINTS

The larger a class is, the more "its" you should have so that all students have an opportunity to be chased. This also gives more children a chance to be "it."

If the same students keep getting tagged, give some other students a chance to be "it."

Watch for children who stay on the Blarney stones for a long time. Set a time limit. Tell them they must run if you think they have been there too long.

At the end of the game, ask the students how many times they were tagged.

A Reel Jig

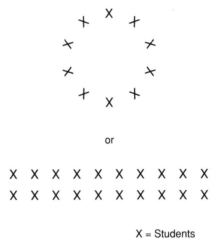

or

X = Students

Figure 6.7 A reel jig.

QUICK DESCRIPTION
Folk dance (Figure 6.7)

APPROPRIATE GRADES
K-6

ACTIVITY GOALS
To perform the dance correctly and to improve the ability to work in a group

SPACE REQUIRED
Gymnasium

KEY SKILLS
Sliding, skipping, and hopping to the beat of the music

EQUIPMENT AND PREPARATION
You will need **a record or cassette player** and **a lively Irish song** such as "McNamara's Band." The public library should have a suitable piece of music.

ACTIVITY PROCEDURE
There are three types of Irish folk dances—jigs, hornpipes, and reels. The jigs and hornpipes are characterized by clogging or tapping steps, and the

reels are characterized by shuffling or gliding steps. The Reel Jig is a simple dance I created to include some characteristics of each.

Arrange the students in a single circle with hands at their sides, or in a double line with the students facing one another. There are no partners when the dance is performed in a circle. When the dance is performed in a line, partners stand across from one another.

The dance is performed in 4/4 time.

MEASURES

1-2   Beginning with the left foot, students take seven sliding steps to the left and hold to a count of 8.

3-4   Beginning with the right foot, students take seven sliding steps to the right and hold to a count of 8.

5   Students hop on the left foot while tapping the right foot in front (right leg is extended), hop again on the left foot while crossing the right foot over and tapping (right knee is bent), hop again on the left foot while tapping the right foot in front (right leg is extended), and then jump on both feet. The movement is done quickly: hop/tap, hop/tap, hop/tap, jump.

6   Repeat Measure 5 while hopping on the right foot and tapping with the left foot.

7-8   Repeat Measures 5 and 6.

9-10   Stepping back on the right foot, students take eight skipping steps backwards.

11-12   Beginning with the right foot, students take eight walking/shuffling steps forward.

13-16   Repeat Measures 9 through 12.

The dance continues by repeating Measures 1 through 16.

SAFETY CONSIDERATIONS

To avoid collisions, slow the music down in the beginning and make sure all the students know which direction they should travel.

ADAPTATION SUGGESTIONS

Choose a slower piece of music for the younger children. You can also have them hold hands on the slides to keep the circle or lines together. If some children can't skip backwards, they can walk or shuffle. If they can't do the hop/tap step, they can hop, hop, hop, jump.

TEACHING HINTS

Allow students time to practice sliding and skipping to the music before teaching the dance.

Chapter 7

APRIL

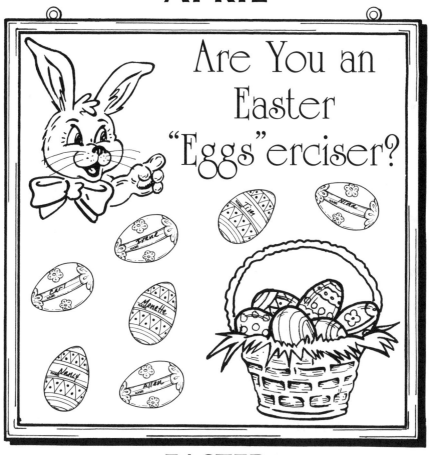

Are You an Easter "Eggs"erciser?

EASTER

Easter "Eggs"ercisers

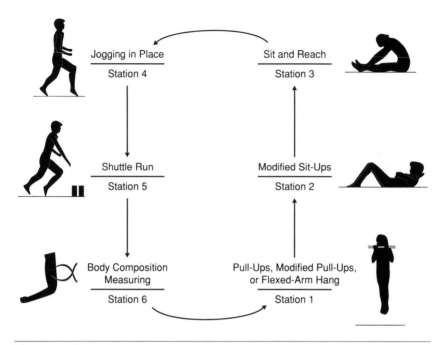

Figure 7.1   I'm an Easter "eggs"erciser.

QUICK DESCRIPTION

Physical fitness exercise circuit training course (Figure 7.1)

APPROPRIATE GRADES

K-6

ACTIVITY GOALS

To improve physical fitness levels, especially muscular strength and endurance and cardiovascular endurance, by motivating the students to put more effort into the physical fitness exercises

SPACE REQUIRED

Gymnasium, track, or large outside area

KEY SKILLS

The April circuit training course emphasizes the following skills and physical fitness tests:

- Arm and shoulder girdle strength (pull-ups, modified pull-ups, flexed-arm hang)

- Abdominal strength and endurance (modified sit-ups)
- Lower back and hamstring flexibility (sit and reach)
- Cardiovascular endurance (jogging in place)
- Agility (shuttle run)
- Body composition measuring or another test such as the standing long jump to test leg power

EQUIPMENT AND PREPARATION

Start this circuit training course at the beginning of April. For the sample circuit training course, construct **7 signs**, one for each of the six exercise stations and one that says "Are You an Easter 'Eggs'erciser?" The station signs should be "Pull-Ups, Modified Pull-Ups, or Flexed-Arm Hang," "Modified Sit-Ups," "Sit and Reach," "Jogging in Place," "Shuttle Run," and "Body Composition Measuring." Reproduce enough **paper "Easter 'Eggs'erciser" certificates** (Figure A.14 in the appendix) for everyone in your class.

Attach the "Are You an Easter 'Eggs'erciser?" sign to a prominent wall or bulletin board along with some **other Easter decorations**. You will also need **1 or 2 pull-up bars, 1 sit-and-reach box, 1 tumbling mat, 8 blocks of wood or chalkboard erasers**, and **skinfold calipers**.

Build excitement and interest by putting up signs around the school about a week before the course is held that say "Easter 'Eggs'ercisers Will Hop to It in Physical Education Class!"

ACTIVITY PROCEDURE

Review the activity procedures for circuit training courses on page xii. Because you will be using Station 6 to measure body composition, the time limit will depend on how long it takes you to measure each student's tricep and calf.

Students earn a paper "Easter 'Eggs'erciser" certificate the first time they complete the course, and a smiling bunny face drawn on the certificate each time after that.

SAFETY CONSIDERATIONS

Emphasize that students use correct form while performing the exercises.

ADAPTATION SUGGESTIONS

Substitute any test for a skill you would like the students to practice.

TEACHING HINTS

Use one of the stations to administer other fitness tests, such as pull-ups, modified sit-ups, sit and reach, and shuttle run. For the body-composition test, tell students to have their right shirt sleeves and right pant legs already rolled up.

Peter Cottontail's Bunny Trail

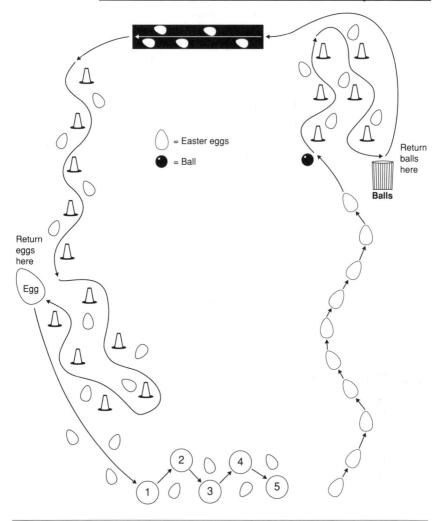

Figure 7.2 Peter Cottontail's bunny trail.

QUICK DESCRIPTION

Obstacle course (Figure 7.2)

APPROPRIATE GRADES

K-6

ACTIVITY GOALS

To perform the skills in the obstacle course correctly without touching any Easter eggs

SPACE REQUIRED

Gymnasium

KEY SKILLS

Bodily control while performing the entire obstacle course, perceptual motor skills, and animal walks

EQUIPMENT AND PREPARATION

Reproduce about **20 paper Easter eggs** (Figure A.15a in the appendix) or cut them out of different-colored pieces of construction paper. Also reproduce enough **"Peter Cottontail Hopped Through It"** certificates (Figure A.15b in the appendix) for everyone in your class. Assemble the obstacle course. You will need **17 traffic cones** or other obstacles, **3 playground balls, 2 tumbling mats**, and **masking tape**.

Motivate the students by putting up signs around the school about a week before the activity begins that say "Will You Be Able to Hop Through Peter Cottontail's Trail?" or "Can You Follow the Bunny Trail Without Stepping on Any Eggs?"

ACTIVITY PROCEDURE

Review the activity procedures for obstacle courses on page xiii. Explain the obstacle course. Students who complete the course correctly without touching any eggs receive a "Peter Cottontail Hopped Through It" certificate.

These activities are included in the sample course:

- Rabbit jumping over eggs on the floor
- Kangaroo jumping through traffic cones
- Seal walking across the mats
- Lame dog walking through traffic cones
- Crab walking while balancing a paper egg on the abdomen
- Hopping from one spot to another without touching the floor with the non-hopping foot

SAFETY CONSIDERATIONS

Emphasize that students start on the signal and stop when they complete the course.

ADAPTATION SUGGESTIONS

Adjust the difficulty of the activities according to skill levels.

TEACHING HINTS

Students should return the playground ball to the starting position after performing the kangaroo jump.

April and Easter Skills Stations

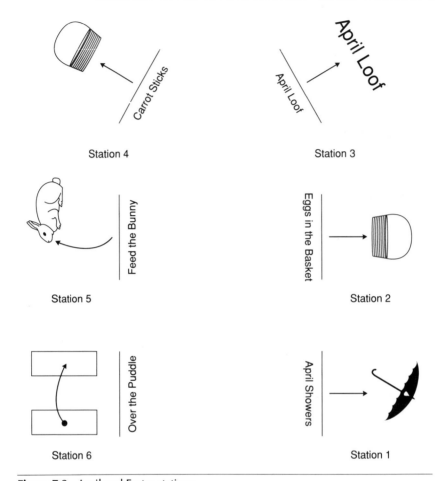

Figure 7.3 April and Easter stations.

QUICK DESCRIPTION
Ball-handling and striking skills stations (Figure 7.3)

APPROPRIATE GRADES
K-6

ACTIVITY GOALS
To improve skill level in rolling, throwing, and striking

SPACE REQUIRED
Gymnasium

KEY SKILLS

Rolling, underhand throwing, overhand throwing, and striking with a hockey stick

EQUIPMENT AND PREPARATION

You will need to do the following for the six stations:

• *April Showers*—Make **a sign** that says "April Showers" and **a large paper raindrop**. Tape the raindrop to an open **umbrella**. You will also need **a sponge or fleece ball**.

• *Eggs in the Basket*—Make **a sign** that says "Eggs in the Basket." You will also need **a small, unbreakable Easter egg or a small ball**, and **a small basket**.

• *April Loof*—Make **a sign** that says "April Loof" ("Fool" is purposely spelled backwards). You will also need **2 beanbags**.

• *Carrot Sticks*—Make **a sign** that says "Carrot Sticks." You will also need **a lummi stick or other small stick**, and **a small basket**.

• *Feed the Bunny*—Make **a sign** that says "Feed the Bunny." You will also need **a large picture of a bunny** and **a beanbag**.

• *Over the Puddle*—Make **a sign** that says "Over the Puddle." You will also need **2 tumbling mats, 1 floor hockey stick**, and **1 hockey puck**.

Set up the stations.

ACTIVITY PROCEDURE

Review the activity procedures for skills stations on page xiv. Explain each station to the class.

Station Description

• *April Showers*—Students hit the paper raindrop, which is attached to the umbrella, using an overhand throw with a sponge or fleece ball.

• *Eggs in the Basket*—Students roll an unbreakable egg or small ball into a basket turned on its side.

• *April Loof*—Students use an overhand throw to hit the letters in the word *fool* in the correct order.

• *Carrot Sticks*—Students use an underhand throw to toss the lummi sticks in the basket.

• *Feed the Bunny*—Students throw overhand trying to hit the bunny's mouth.

• *Over the Puddle*—Students hit the hockey puck from one mat so it goes over the "puddle" (the space between the two mats) and lands on the other mat.

SAFETY CONSIDERATIONS

Tell the students to keep the hockey stick close to the floor. Emphasize that the hockey puck won't land on the other mat if it is hit too hard. Stress control.

ADAPTATION SUGGESTIONS

Shorten or lengthen the distance from the throwing line to the target depending on skill level.

TEACHING HINTS

Teach the skills to the students before they practice at the stations. Stress correct form when they are performing the skills.

Easter "Eggs"ercise Hunt

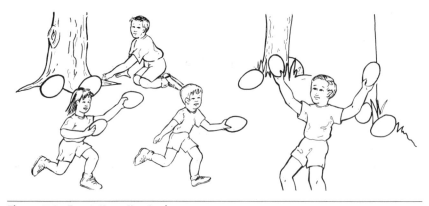

Figure 7.4 Easter "eggs"ercise hunt.

QUICK DESCRIPTION

Exercise game and Easter egg hunt (Figure 7.4)

APPROPRIATE GRADES

K-6

ACTIVITY GOALS

To learn the names of the exercises and to perform them correctly

SPACE REQUIRED

Outside area

KEY SKILLS

Performing selected exercises. (Sharing the hidden eggs is also an important part of this lesson.)

EQUIPMENT AND PREPARATION

Make enough **paper Easter eggs from construction paper** so that each student in the class can find five. On each egg, write the name of an exercise the students have performed throughout the year. You can write the same exercise on more than one egg.

ACTIVITY PROCEDURE

Have some older students hide the eggs for your classes or have the previous class hide them. Show the students a sample of the egg used in the hunt. Tell them that you have hidden enough eggs so everyone can find five. The students should not pick up more than five eggs. On the signal, students begin looking for the eggs. When they find five, they return to the exercise area. When the whole class has returned, have them space themselves out and then say the name of one of the exercises. Students who have this exercise on one of their eggs come up to the front of the class and lead the class in that exercise. Keep calling out exercises until everyone has had a turn to lead. If someone's exercises were not called, have them choose one from their eggs and lead the class. When class is over, collect the eggs or have the students hide the eggs for the next class.

SAFETY CONSIDERATIONS

Emphasize correct form while the students are performing the exercises.

Show students the area where the eggs are hidden so they don't wander off trying to find them.

ADAPTATION SUGGESTIONS

You can write other activities on the eggs, such as locomotor skills, stunts, and movement challenges.

TEACHING HINTS

Choose exercises with which the children are familiar.

Peter Cottontail Tag

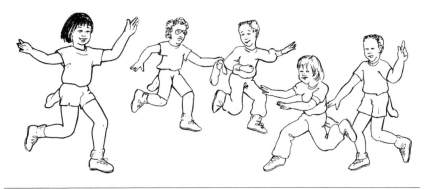

Figure 7.5 Peter Cottontail tag.

QUICK DESCRIPTION

A chasing and fleeing game (Figure 7.5)

APPROPRIATE GRADES

K-6

ACTIVITY GOALS

To demonstrate bodily control and knowledge of game and safety rules in a game situation

SPACE REQUIRED

Gymnasium or outside area with marked boundaries

KEY SKILLS

Running, chasing, fleeing, and dodging; and developing honesty and good sportsmanship

EQUIPMENT AND PREPARATION

You will need **a tail** (a sock or flag-football flag) **for each student in the class**. If you use socks as the tails, ask the students to bring old white socks to school. Mark off boundaries if necessary. You might need traffic cones to do this.

ACTIVITY PROCEDURE

Give students a "tail." Show them how to tuck one end of it into their pants waistbands or their belt loops. If they do not have waistbands or belt loops, have them tuck the tail in the back part of the neckline or in the sleeve of their shirts or dresses. Every player is a chaser and is being chased simultaneously. When you give the signal, students try to pull out as many of the other players' tails as they can while preventing their own tails from being pulled out. Players may touch only the tails, not the players. If a player touches the other player when taking a tail, the other player keeps his or her tail until someone pulls it out correctly. Students may continue to play after their tails have been pulled out. The last one left with a tail or the player who has pulled out the most tails is the winner. You can decide which way you want the students to play.

SAFETY CONSIDERATIONS

Emphasize that students pull the tails gently and don't grab another player's clothing or body.

Clear the playing area of hazards and keep the boundary lines away from walls or fences to avoid accidents. Also stress that the students watch where they are running at all times to avoid collisions.

ADAPTATION SUGGESTIONS

Reduce the size of the playing area for younger children.

TEACHING HINTS

Watch for the child who sometimes hides the tail and pulls it out later in the game when only a small number of players have tails left.

Scrambled Eggs

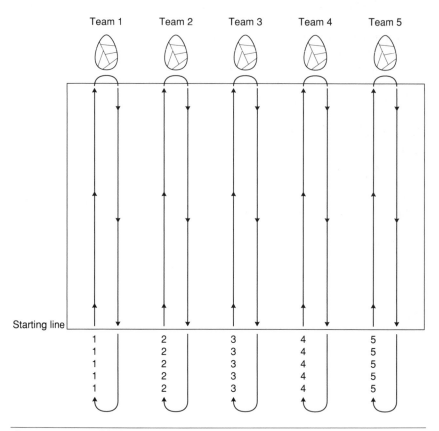

Figure 7.6 Scrambled eggs.

QUICK DESCRIPTION
Cooperative relay race (Figure 7.6)

APPROPRIATE GRADES
K-6

ACTIVITY GOALS
To perform the locomotor skills correctly, work cooperatively in a group, and demonstrate knowledge of game and safety rules in a game situation

SPACE REQUIRED
Gymnasium

KEY SKILLS

Various locomotor skills, such as running, galloping, skipping, and animal walks; participating cooperatively in a group; obeying the rules of a game; and demonstrating knowledge of safety rules while playing a game

EQUIPMENT AND PREPARATION

Cut out **4 or 5 large paper Easter eggs**, laminate them, and cut them into puzzles. You can have older students make these for you. Have them decorate one side of the egg and leave the other side blank. It would be too difficult for the students to unscramble the pieces with the egg decorated on both sides. The number of egg puzzles will depend on the number of relay teams you will have. Cut each of the eggs equally into pieces so there is at least one piece for every student on each team. You will also need **a small container for each puzzle** (turned-over flying disks work fine).

ACTIVITY PROCEDURE

Explain the relay race to the class. Divide the class, as evenly as possible, into four or five relay teams. Arrange the teams in single-file lines at one end of the gym behind a starting line. Make a line with masking tape if there's no line on the gym floor. At the other end of the gym, place a container with the puzzle pieces even with each team. To avoid confusion, make sure each team knows its container. It's a good idea to walk each team through the race procedure first. On the signal, the first student in each line performs the designated locomotor skill while approaching the container, takes one piece of the puzzle from the container, returns to the starting line, and tags right hands with the next team member. This procedure continues until all of the puzzle pieces have been retrieved from the container. As the race is in progress, team members work to put the puzzle pieces together. The first team to finish the puzzle correctly, wins. Teams can exchange puzzles and race again.

SAFETY CONSIDERATIONS

Place the starting line and containers a safe distance from walls to avoid accidents. Also, stress that students tag right hands to avoid collisions. Don't allow the students to slide to the finish line.

ADAPTATION SUGGESTIONS

Vary the locomotor skills according to ability. You can make the puzzle more difficult by not decorating it. However, do mark each piece on one side or it will be too difficult. The marked side should face the floor when the students put the puzzle together.

TEACHING HINTS

This is a good relay because a team that is lagging behind due to the speed of the students' locomotor skills can still win if it puts the puzzle together quickly. Stress cooperation.

Bunny Hop

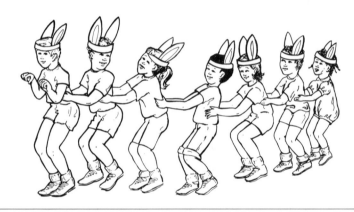

Figure 7.7   Bunny hop.

QUICK DESCRIPTION

A line dance (Figure 7.7)

APPROPRIATE GRADES

K-6

ACTIVITY GOALS

To perform the dance correctly and to improve the ability to work cooperatively in a group

SPACE REQUIRED

Gymnasium

KEY SKILLS

Jumping to the beat of the music

EQUIPMENT AND PREPARATION

You will need **a record or cassette player** and **a recording of the "Bunny Hop."** You should be able to find it at the public library.

ACTIVITY PROCEDURE

Play part of the music so the students become familiar with it.
The dance is performed in 4/4 time.

MEASURES

1   Students touch the right heel out to the side, and then touch the right toe near the left foot. Repeat.

2   Students touch the left heel out to the side, and then touch the left toe near the right foot. Repeat.

3-4   Students jump forward and hold, jump backward and hold, and take three quick jumps forward.

The dance continues by repeating Measures 1-4. First teach the dance steps without the music. Then have the students perform the steps to the music. When they are performing the steps correctly and in time to the music, arrange the students in a single-file line. Have the students perform the steps without the music and then with the music. When they are doing the steps correctly, have the students hold onto the shoulders or waist of the person in front of them. Have them perform the dance again without and with the music. If your class is large, you may want to divide the students into several lines. The leader leads the line in any direction around the gym.

SAFETY CONSIDERATIONS

Stress that the students take small jumps. All students should be performing the steps correctly before doing the dance in a single-file line while holding onto shoulders or waists. Students will bump and step on each other if they aren't synchronized. The line leaders must be careful not to collide with the other lines.

ADAPTATION SUGGESTIONS

The "Bunny Hop" is quite lively. You may have to slow it down for the younger children.

TEACHING HINTS

Make sure that the students know the difference between hopping and jumping. Even though the dance is called the "Bunny Hop," the step performed in the dance is actually a jump with both feet (hopping is done on one foot). Younger students can make bunny-ear headbands to wear when they perform the dance. You could also have an Easter bunny costume. To reward some of the older students, allow them to take turns wearing the costume and doing the "Bunny Hop" with the younger classes.

Chapter 8

MAY/JUNE

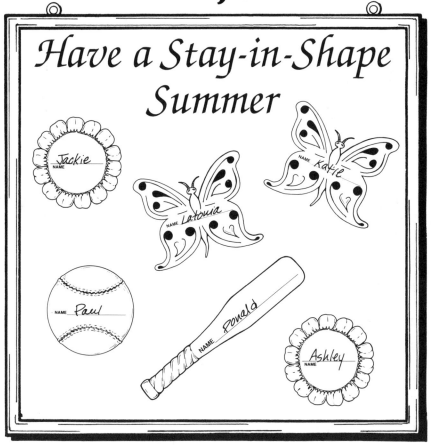

Have a Stay-in-Shape Summer

SUMMER ACTIVITIES

Summer Stay-in-Shape Selections

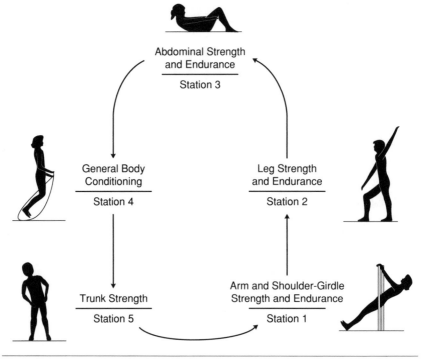

Figure 8.1 Summer stay-in-shape stations.

QUICK DESCRIPTION

Physical fitness exercise circuit training course (Figure 8.1)

APPROPRIATE GRADES

K-6

ACTIVITY GOALS

To improve physical fitness levels, especially cardiovascular endurance, by motivating the students to put more effort into the physical fitness exercises, and to review exercises so students can exercise throughout the summer

SPACE REQUIRED

Gymnasium, track, or large outside area

KEY SKILLS

To review muscular strength and endurance exercises and to improve muscular strength and endurance and cardiovascular endurance

EQUIPMENT AND PREPARATION

Start this circuit training course at the beginning of May. For the sample circuit training course, you will need **the exercise signs** for the exercises the students have learned during the year. Organize the signs according to the muscle groups being exercised and attach the signs to the wall. For example, group all of the exercises that develop arm and shoulder-girdle strength and endurance at one station, and all of the abdominal strength and endurance exercises together at another station. The other stations would include leg strength and endurance, trunk strength, and general body conditioning.

Make **a sign for each station** (e.g., "Arm and Shoulder-Girdle Strength and Endurance"). You will need to reproduce enough **paper flowers** (Figure A.16a in the appendix), **butterflies** (Figure A.16b in the appendix), **baseballs** (Figure A.16c in the appendix), and **baseball bats** (Figure A.16d in the appendix) for everyone in your class.

Also make **a sign** that says "Have a Stay-in-Shape Summer!" Attach the sign to a wall or bulletin board where everyone can see it, and set up the exercise stations. You will also need **a few sets of hand weights, exercise rubber bands**, and **some jump ropes**.

Build excitement and interest by putting up signs around the school about a week before the event is held that say "Will You Remember to Stay in Shape Over the Summer?" or "Choose Your Favorite Exercises From Physical Education Class."

ACTIVITY PROCEDURE

Review the activity procedures for circuit training courses on page xii. Allow 15 to 20 seconds at the stations.

Students earn a paper flower, butterfly, baseball, or baseball bat the first time they correctly complete the course. Draw a sunshine face on it each time they correctly complete the course after that.

SAFETY CONSIDERATIONS

Emphasize that students use correct form while performing the exercises. Tell the students to clear the jogging area of equipment when they are finished.

ADAPTATION SUGGESTIONS

Students can choose different exercises each time they participate in the course. They can also perform different locomotor skills, such as galloping or skipping, each time they change stations.

TEACHING HINTS

To motivate the students to exercise over summer vacation, give them a list of the exercises and tell them to keep a record of which exercises they perform, the number of times they perform them, and how often they perform them. Give some type of reward to students who exercise and keep a record, and whose parents verify that they have done so by signing their record sheet.

Lost While on Summer Vacation

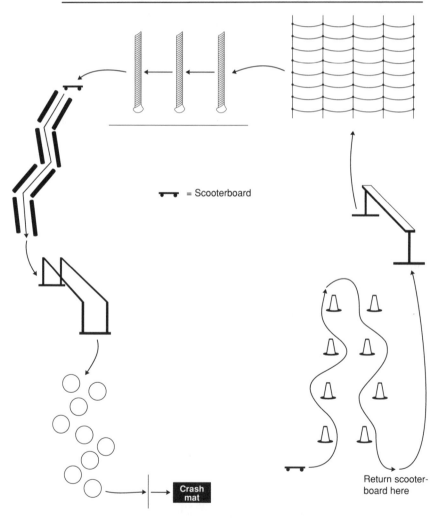

Figure 8.2   Lost while on summer vacation.

QUICK DESCRIPTION
Obstacle course (Figure 8.2)

APPROPRIATE GRADES
K-6

ACTIVITY GOALS
To complete the skills in the obstacle course correctly with a maximum of five errors

SPACE REQUIRED
Gymnasium

KEY SKILLS
Demonstrating bodily control while performing the entire obstacle course; using perceptual motor skills; performing various locomotor skills on the balance beam; traveling from one hanging rope to another; maneuvering through obstacles on the scooterboards while sitting or lying in a prone position; climbing a cargo net; climbing over obstacles; and leaping

EQUIPMENT AND PREPARATION
Reproduce enough **"I Found My Way Home" certificates** (Figure A.17 in the appendix) for everyone in your class.

Assemble the obstacle course. You will need some or all of the following: **1 low balance beam, 8 Hula Hoops or tires, hanging ropes, 1 cargo net, parallel bars or 1 horizontal ladder, 4 folding tumbling mats, 8 traffic cones, 4 scooterboards**, and **1 or 2 crash mats**.

Build excitement and interest by putting up signs around the school about a week before the course is performed that say "Will You Find Your Way Home or Be Lost Forever?" or "Will You Make It Home Through the Quicksand, Wild Animals, and Alligators? You'll Find Out Soon in Physical Education Class."

ACTIVITY PROCEDURE
Review the activity procedures for obstacle courses on page xiii. Explain the obstacle course. Students who complete the course correctly receive an "I Found My Way Home" certificate.

These activities are included in the sample obstacle course:

• *Swim to Safety*—Students maneuver scooterboards through traffic cones while lying in a prone (face down) position. Touching a cone is an error.

• *Hungry Alligators*—Students skip across the balance beam. Falling off before making it all the way across is an error.

- *Climb the Mountain*—Students climb the cargo net to a designated height and climb down. Not climbing to the designated height is an error and jumping off before climbing all the way down is an error.

- *Quicksand*—Students travel from one hanging rope to another without touching the mat. Touching the mat before finishing is an error.

- *Canoe Paddling*—Students sit on a scooterboard and maneuver it through a maze of folding mats standing on their edges. Touching the mats is an error.

- *Escape From the Wild Animals*—Students travel across parallel bars or a horizontal ladder in any safe way. Touching the mat before completely crossing is an error.

- *Helpful Turtles*—Students pretend Hula Hoops or tires are turtles who let them stand on their backs. Students leap from one to another. Stepping on a hoop is an error.

- *Home Sweet Home*—After completing all seven stations, students perform a standing long jump from behind a line to a crash mat, which they can pretend is their bed at home.

SAFETY CONSIDERATIONS

Emphasize that the students start on the signal and stop when they have completed the course.

ADAPTATION SUGGESTIONS

Vary the activities according to the skill level. Limit the climbing height on the cargo net for younger children. They may also need some help transferring from one hanging rope to another.

TEACHING HINTS

Choose activities with which the children are familiar.

The more interesting and exciting you make the story that goes along with the obstacle course, the more the children will love it.

Summer Skills Stations

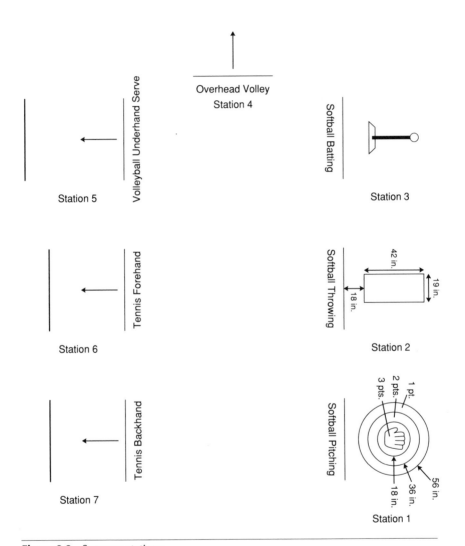

Figure 8.3 Summer stations.

QUICK DESCRIPTION

Summer activity skills stations (Figure 8.3)

APPROPRIATE GRADES

K-6

ACTIVITY GOALS

To improve form and accuracy while throwing and pitching a softball, batting, performing a volleyball serve and an overhead volley, and performing forehand and backhand strokes with a racket

SPACE REQUIRED

Gymnasium or outside area with walls

KEY SKILLS

Softball overhand throw, softball pitch or underhand throw, softball batting, volleyball overhead volley, volleyball underhand serve, tennis forehand stroke, and tennis backhand stroke

EQUIPMENT AND PREPARATION

You will need **a picture of a softball glove**. You can probably find one in an equipment catalog or an older student can draw one for you. You will also need **2 lines on the wall the height of a tennis net** and **2 lines the height of a volleyball net**. Put tape on the wall for **a strike-zone pitching target** (42 inches long and 19 inches wide with the bottom line of the target 18 inches from the floor). Also tape **a throwing target** to the wall (three concentric circles of 18, 36, and 56 inches with the picture of the glove in the center of the 18-inch circle).

Make **7 signs**, one for each station. The signs should be "Softball Pitching," "Softball Throwing," "Softball Batting," "Overhead Volley," "Volleyball Underhand Serve," "Tennis Forehand," and "Tennis Backhand." Set up the stations. You will also need **3 softballs, 1 batting tee, 2 volleyballs or beachballs, 2 tennis rackets**, and **2 tennis balls**.

ACTIVITY PROCEDURE

Review the activity procedures for skills stations on page xiv. Explain each station to the class.

Station Description

(Students can keep score if desired)

• *Softball Overhand Throw*—Students use an overhand throw to hit the softball glove picture. A direct hit is worth 3 points, the outside circle is worth 1 point, and the middle circle is worth 2 points.

• *Softball Pitch*—Students use an underhand softball pitch to hit inside the strike zone taped to the wall. One point is earned if the ball hits within the target.

• *Softball Batting*—Students hit the ball off the batting tee. One point is earned if they hit the ball correctly.

- *Volleyball Overhead Volley*—Students volley the ball three consecutive times over the line taped to the wall. One point is earned if they do this correctly.

- *Volleyball Underhand Serve*—Students serve the ball so it hits the wall above the line taped to the wall. One point is earned if they do this correctly.

- *Tennis Forehand Stroke*—Students hit the ball above the line taped to the wall using a forehand stroke. One point is earned if they do this correctly.

- *Tennis Backhand Stroke*—Students hit the ball above the line taped to the wall using a backhand stroke. One point is earned if they do this correctly.

SAFETY CONSIDERATIONS

Leave ample space between the stations. Stress that the students stand away from the person taking a turn so they don't get hit accidentally, especially at the batting and tennis stations.

ADAPTATION SUGGESTIONS

For the younger children you can use a lightweight plastic bat and ball instead of a softball bat and ball. You can also use beachballs instead of volleyballs.

Adjust the distance from the restraining line to the targets according to skill level.

Older students will enjoy keeping score.

TEACHING HINTS

Students should have had some previous experience with the skills before this station lesson.

Hot-Weather Water Tag

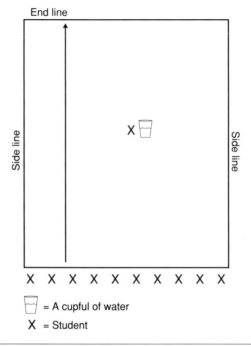

Figure 8.4 Hot-weather water tag.

QUICK DESCRIPTION
A chasing and fleeing game with no bodily contact (Figure 8.4)

APPROPRIATE GRADES
K-6

ACTIVITY GOALS
To demonstrate bodily control and knowledge of game and safety rules in a game situation

SPACE REQUIRED
Outside area (preferably grass)

KEY SKILLS
Running, chasing, fleeing, and dodging

EQUIPMENT AND PREPARATION

Mark off a large playing area with two end lines and two side lines. You might need traffic cones for this. Find **a source of water** near your outside playing area. Fill **1 or 2 buckets** with water and provide **1 small plastic or paper cup for each student** (the soft plastic kind hold up best).

ACTIVITY PROCEDURE

Line up the entire class along one of the end lines. Pick one of the students to be "it" and have him or her stand in the center of the playing area (beside the buckets of water). Give this student a small cup of water to hold. The game begins when the person who is "it" says "It's time to cool off." This is the signal for the other players to run to the other end line while trying to avoid getting the cup of water thrown on them. Once the signal has been given, the players are not safe until they reach the other end line. If they stay on the starting end line, they can be splashed. Players who get splashed are considered "tagged" and during the next round become helpers of the person who is "it." All the helpers stand in the center of the playing area with a small cup of water and give the starting signal: "It's time to cool off." The players once again run to the other end line, trying to avoid getting wet. This procedure repeats until there is only one "dry" player left. This player becomes "it" in the next game.

SAFETY CONSIDERATIONS

Use very small cups of water and emphasize that students throw the water below the neck, not in the face.

ADAPTATION SUGGESTIONS

You might want to have more than one player be "it" and start a new game when there are three "dry" players left.

TEACHING HINTS

Watch for students who play with the water and get wetter than one should from just playing the game. Save this game for a day when the classroom teacher won't mind if the students get a little wet.

Fill It Up

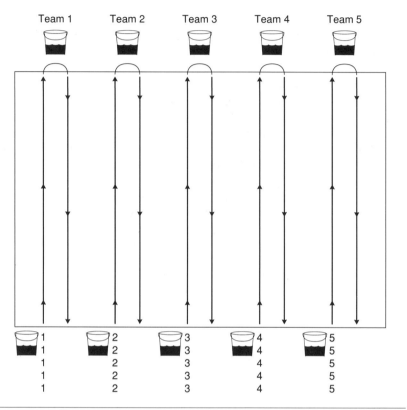

Team 1   Team 2   Team 3   Team 4   Team 5

```
1         2         3         4         5
1         2         3         4         5
1         2         3         4         5
1         2         3         4         5
1         2         3         4         5
```

Figure 8.5 Fill it up.

QUICK DESCRIPTION

An aerobic water-transferring team race (Figure 8.5)

APPROPRIATE GRADES

K-6

ACTIVITY GOALS

To run or walk fast continually, work cooperatively in a group, and demonstrate knowledge of game and safety rules in a game situation

SPACE REQUIRED

Outside area (preferably grass)

KEY SKILLS

Endurance running and following game and safety rules

EQUIPMENT AND PREPARATION

You will need **2 buckets or containers for each team, 1 measuring cup**, and **a very small plastic or paper cup for each student** (the soft plastic cups hold up best). Find **a source of water** near the outside playing area, and fill one bucket for each team.

ACTIVITY PROCEDURE

Explain the race to the class. Divide the class, as evenly as possible, into teams. Teams of four or five work well. Arrange each team, single file, at one end of the playing field behind a bucket of water. Place an empty bucket or container at the other end of the playing field even with each team. Make sure each team knows which empty bucket is theirs. Give each student a small cup. On the signal, all of the students fill their cups with water from the bucket in front of them, run to the empty bucket, pour in the water from their cups, and run back to the starting bucket and fill their cups again.

As long as there are only four or five on each team, it works well for all the students to run at once—they'll experience the benefits of continuous aerobic exercise. Just make sure to leave space between the teams, to avoid collisions. Students may place one hand over the top of their cup to prevent the water from spilling when they run. Students repeat this procedure until the signal is given. Water may not be transferred after the signal. Measure the amount of water in each bucket. The team with the most water is the winner. Adjust the time limit for the game according to the students' abilities.

SAFETY CONSIDERATIONS

To avoid collisions, tell students to watch where they are running and to keep to the right. Also warn students that the grass might become a little wet and slippery.

ADAPTATION SUGGESTIONS

Adjust the distance between buckets according to ability. You can also adjust the time limit.

TEACHING HINTS

This race gives the students a good aerobic workout by motivating them to run continuously. They are so busy filling the buckets that they don't notice how much they are running.

The measuring of the water at the end of the race can become a math lesson if you use a graded measuring cup. It also seems more official to the students when the water is accurately measured.

Barefoot and "Marble"ous

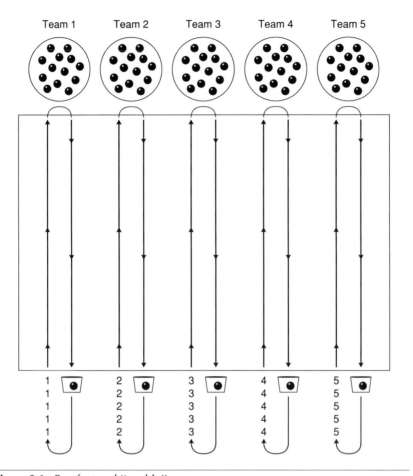

Figure 8.6 Barefoot and "marble"ous.

QUICK DESCRIPTION

A marble-transferring relay using only the feet (Figure 8.6)

APPROPRIATE GRADES

K-6

ACTIVITY GOALS

To manipulate marbles with the feet, work cooperatively in a group, and demonstrate knowledge of game and safety rules in a game situation

SPACE REQUIRED

Gymnasium or large classroom

KEY SKILLS

Manipulating objects with the feet, and following game and safety rules

EQUIPMENT AND PREPARATION

Each team will need **12 or more marbles, a Hula Hoop, a container** (flying disks turned over work great), and **a few pieces of masking tape**. Tape one hoop to the floor at the end of the playing area opposite each team, and place an equal number of marbles in each.

ACTIVITY PROCEDURE

Explain the relay to the class. Divide the class, as evenly as possible, into relay teams. The students will get more turns if the teams are small (four or five students). Have the students take off their shoes and socks. Arrange each team, single file, behind one of the containers at one end of the gym. Make sure each team knows which hoop is their's. On the signal, the first student in each line runs to the hoop, picks up one marble (only one is allowed each time) with the toes, and runs, hops, or performs any other locomotor movement back to the starting line. The student then releases the marble from the toes into the container and goes to the end of the line. The next student in line repeats the same procedure. This student must wait until the marble is deposited in the container before he or she can run. Students keep taking turns until all of the marbles have been transferred from the Hula Hoop to the container. If a student loses control of a marble, he or she must retrieve it using the feet only. The team that transfers all of the marbles from the hoop to the container first is the winner.

SAFETY CONSIDERATIONS

Make sure the gym floor is clean, and clear of any foreign objects that might injure a student. Also clear away any chairs or tables so there is no possibility of students stubbing their toes. Have the students put their shoes in a designated spot, away from the playing area. Tape the hoops to the floor to prevent them from slipping.

ADAPTATION SUGGESTIONS

Adjust the distance from the containers to the hoops, and the number of marbles according to ability.

TEACHING HINTS

If a student loses control of a marble, watch to see that he or she retrieves it with the feet and not the hands. It is awkward using only the feet and some students will accidentally use their hands.

Swim to the Beat

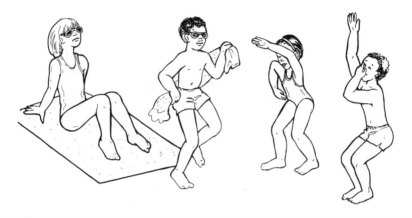

Figure 8.7 Swim to the beat.

QUICK DESCRIPTION

Aerobic dance activity (Figure 8.7)

APPROPRIATE GRADES

K-6

ACTIVITY GOALS

To perform the steps of the dance correctly to the beat of the music, and to raise heart rates to the target zone

SPACE REQUIRED

Gymnasium

KEY SKILLS

Performing arm strokes for the front crawl, back crawl, breaststroke, side-stroke, and butterfly stroke; running, jumping, and hopping; and developing a sense of rhythm

EQUIPMENT AND PREPARATION

You will need **a record or cassette player** and **a lively piece of music** that the students will like. A suggestion is "Here Comes Summer" by Jerry Keller (MCA Records/Jaymar Music Publishing Company).

ACTIVITY PROCEDURE

Have the students scatter on the floor with ample space between them. They should all face the same direction. Choose music in 4/4 time. Play part of the music before you begin teaching the steps to familiarize the students with it. Teach some of the steps without music and then have the students practice the steps to the music. Continue this procedure until all of the steps have been learned.

MEASURES

1-4   Students sit on floor and lean back on the forearms. They flutter-kick legs, alternating legs on each beat.

5-8   Students turn over and lie in a prone position. They flutter-kick legs, alternating legs on each beat.

9-12   Students stand and do the arm stroke of the front crawl while jumping in place. They jump once on each beat.

13-16   Students do the arm stroke of the back crawl while jumping in place. They jump once on each beat.

17-18   Students do the arm stroke of the sidestroke while hopping and stepping to the left. They do one arm stroke for each hop on the left foot and each step on the right foot.

19-20   Students repeat the last sequence while moving to the right (hopping on the right foot and stepping with the left).

21-22   Students repeat action from Measures 17-18.

23-24   Students repeat action from Measures 19-20.

25-28   Students do the arm stroke of the breaststroke while running in place. Alternate feet should hit the floor on each beat.

29-32   Students do the arm stroke of the butterfly stroke while jumping forward. They jump once on each beat.

33-40   Students pretend to dry off with a towel while doing the twist.

Repeat the sequence as many times as desired.

SAFETY CONSIDERATIONS

Make sure the students have enough room between them so they don't accidentally hit each other.

ADAPTATION SUGGESTIONS

You can make movements from other sports into an aerobic dance routine.

TEACHING HINTS

Keep the movements simple so the students can do them continuously and get a good aerobic workout.

To make the routine more creative, have the students wear swimsuits, sunglasses, sunhats, and visors. They can start out by sitting on beach towels so it looks like they are at the beach. During the twisting part, have them pick up their towels and pretend to be drying off.

Appendix A

REPRODUCIBLE AWARDS AND MATERIALS

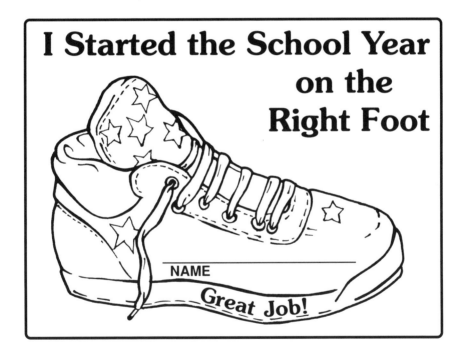

Figure A.1a "I Started the School Year on the Right Foot" certificate.

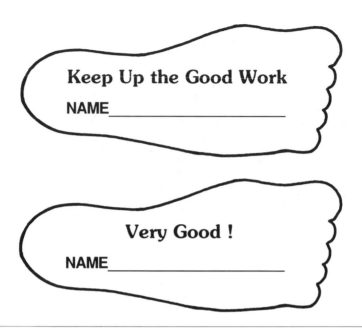

Figure A.1b   Footnotes.

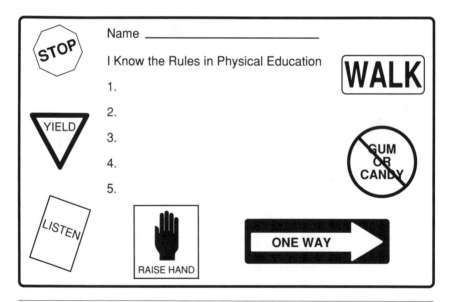

Figure A.2   September obstacle course award.

Monster Muscles

Name _____

Draw your favorite monster above.

Figure A.3a "Monster Muscles" certificate.

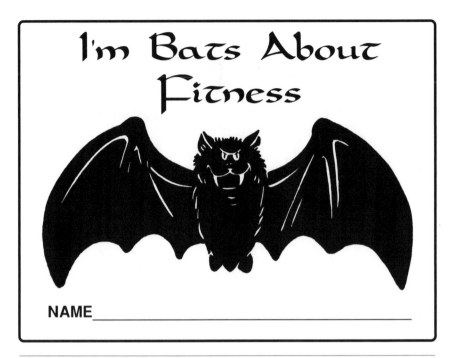

Figure A.3b "I'm Bats About Fitness" certificate.

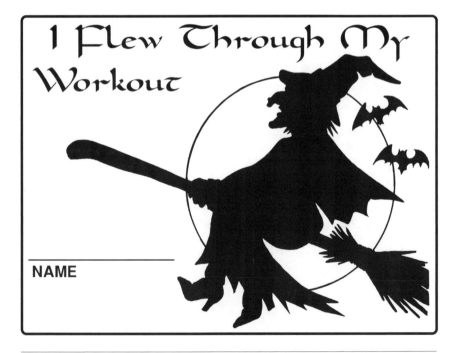

Figure A.3c "I Flew Through My Workout" certificate.

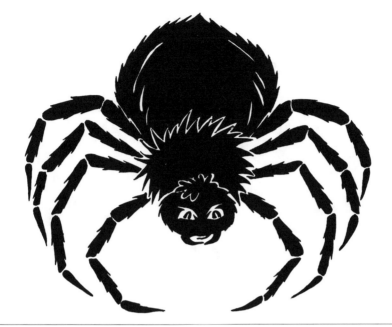

Figure A.4a Spiders to attach to October obstacle course.

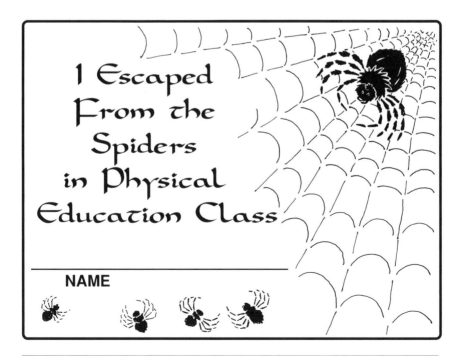

Figure A.4b "I Escaped From the Spiders" award.

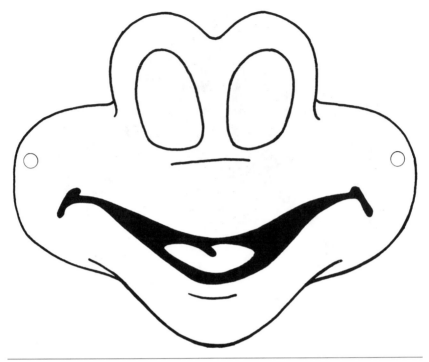

Figure A.5 Frog mask.

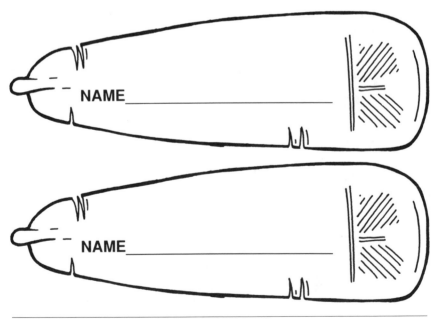

NAME_____

NAME_____

Figure A.6 "Turkey feather" awards.

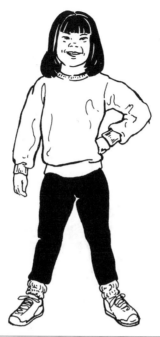

Figure A.7a Paper person to attach to November obstacle course.

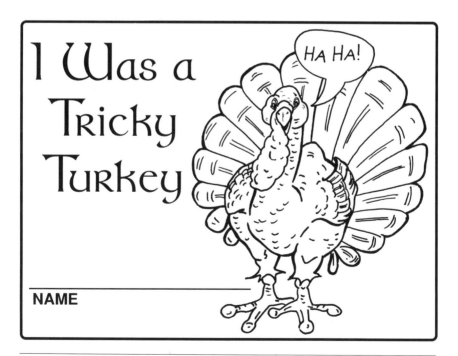

Figure A.7b "I Was a Tricky Turkey" certificate.

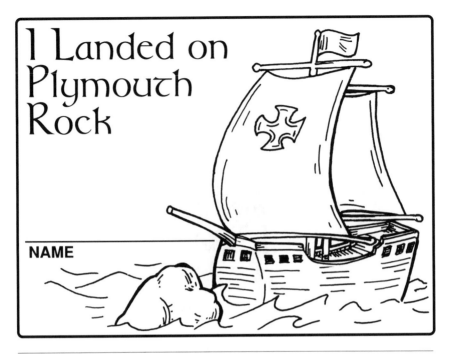

Figure A.7c "I Landed on Plymouth Rock" certificate.

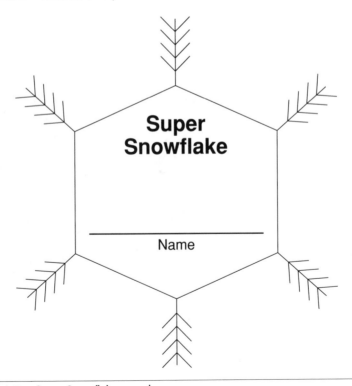

Figure A.8a Super Snowflake award.

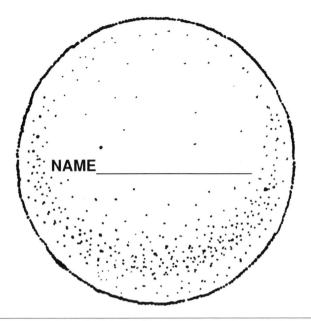

NAME_____

Figure A.8b Snowperson's body award.

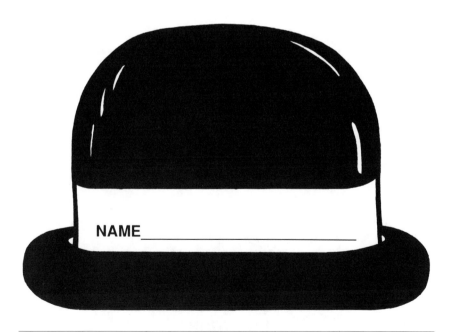

NAME_____

Figure A.8c Snowperson's top hat award.

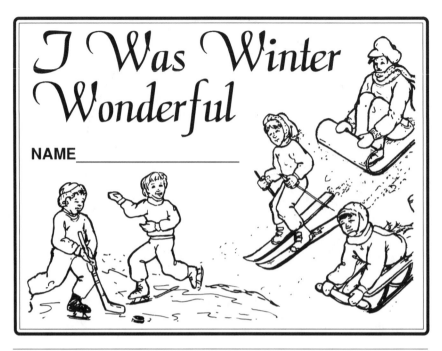

Figure A.9 December/January obstacle course award.

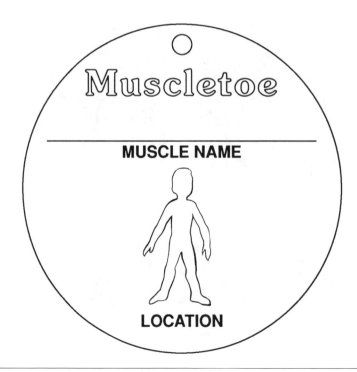

Figure A.10 Muscletoe name and location card.

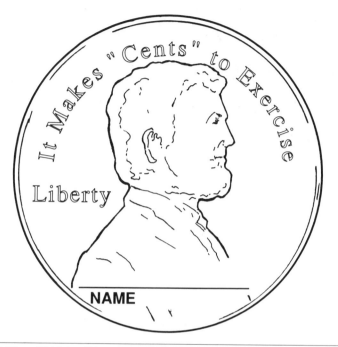

Figure A.11a "It Makes 'Cents' to Exercise" penny certificate.

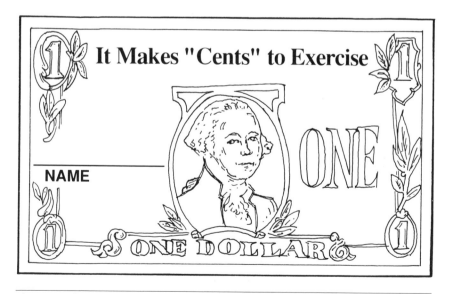

Figure A.11b. "It Makes 'Cents' to Exercise" dollar bill certificate.

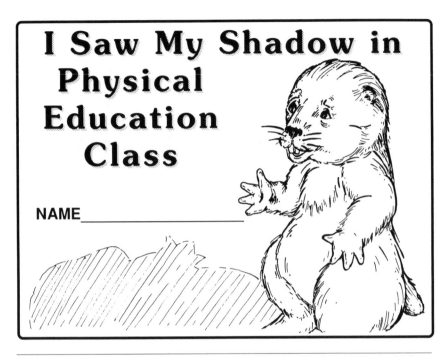

Figure A.12 February obstacle course award: "I Saw My Shadow in Physical Education Class."

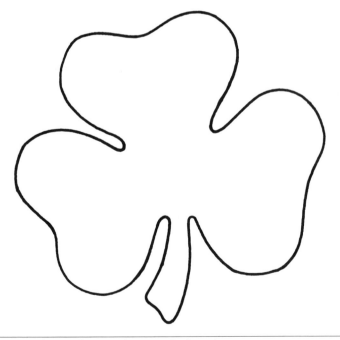

Figure A.13a Shamrock to attach to March obstacle course.

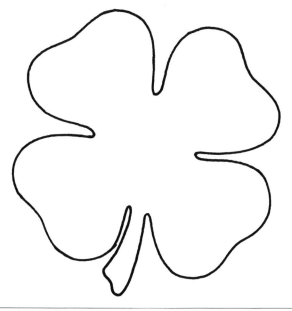

Figure A.13b Four-leaf clover to attach to March obstacle course.

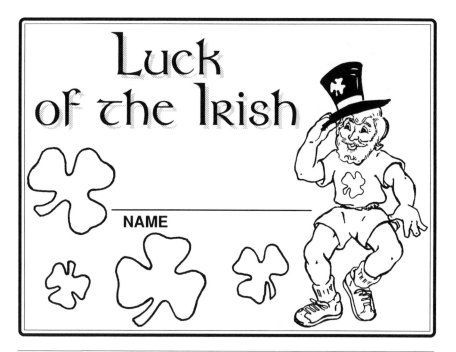

Figure A.13c "Luck of the Irish" certificate.

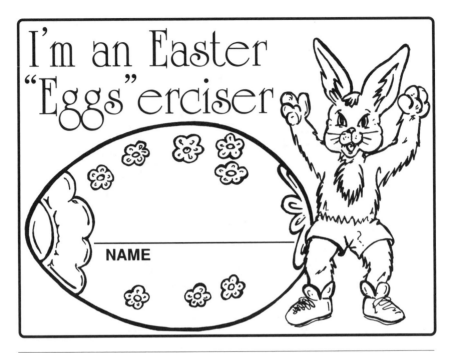

Figure A.14   April circuit training course award: "I'm an Easter 'Eggs'erciser."

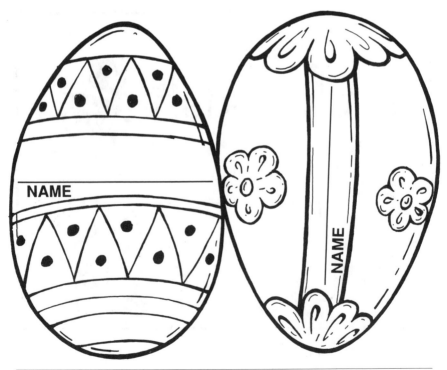

Figure A.15a   Easter eggs to attach to course.

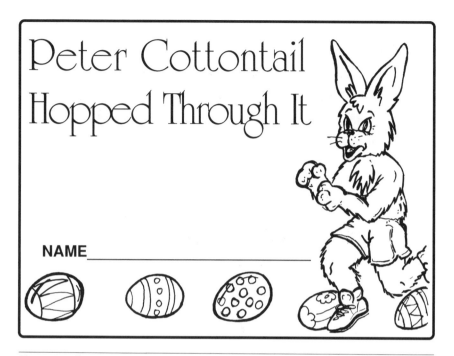

Figure A.15b "Peter Cottontail Hopped Through It" certificate.

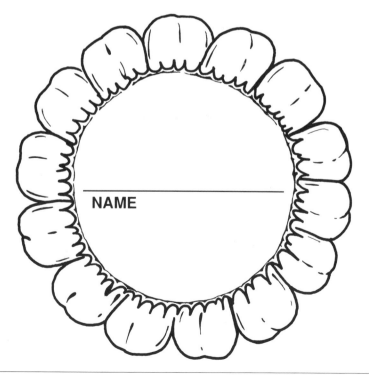

Figure A.16a Flower award.

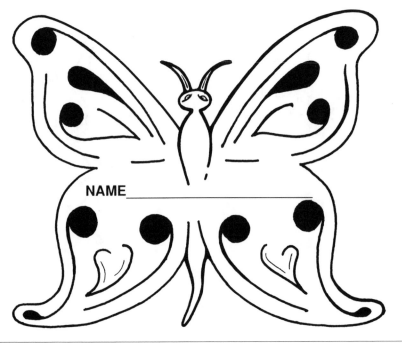

Figure A.16b Butterfly award.

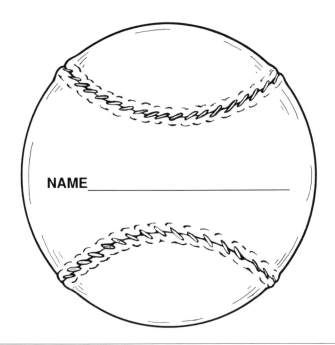

Figure A.16c Baseball award.

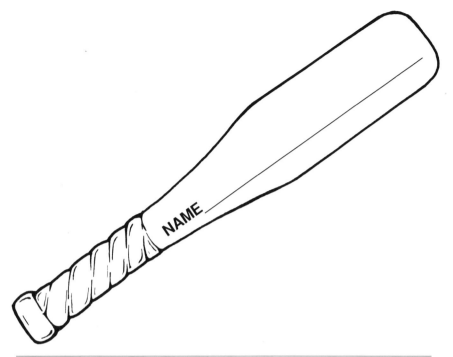

Figure A.16d Baseball bat award.

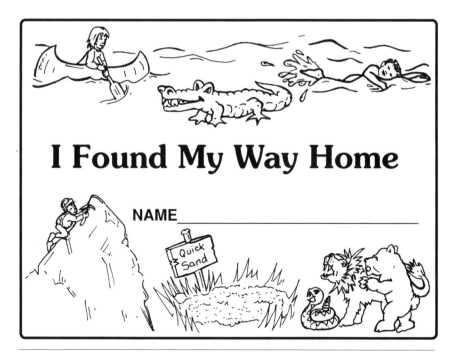

Figure A.17 "I Found My Way Home" certificate.

About the Author

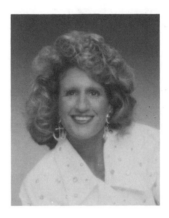

Barbara Wnek developed the fun activities in *Holiday Games and Activities* in her own physical education classes. Since 1977, she has taught children from ages 3 through 14 in both public and private settings. She believes in creating fun, success-oriented learning experiences to help students enjoy physical education.

Barbara currently teaches physical education to kids in elementary school in the Ferguson-Florissant School District near St. Louis, Missouri. During the summer, she serves as the physical education director for the Gifted Resource Council's summer camps, where she creates and teaches physical education activities related to the camps' varying themes. She is also a certified aerobics instructor and an American Red Cross first aid, CPR, and swimming instructor.

Barbara earned her master's degree in elementary education with an emphasis in exercise physiology from the University of Missouri–St. Louis. She is a member of the American Alliance for Health, Physical Education, Recreation and Dance (AAHPERD).